BIOCHEMISTRY AND MOLECULAR BIOLOGY
IN THE POST GENOMIC ERA

BIOCOMPOSITES IN
BIO-MEDICINE

BIOCHEMISTRY AND MOLECULAR BIOLOGY IN THE POST GENOMIC ERA

Additional books and e-books in this series can be found on Nova's website under the Series tab.

NEW DEVELOPMENTS IN MEDICAL RESEARCH

Additional books and e-books in this series can be found on Nova's website under the Series tab.

BIOCHEMISTRY AND MOLECULAR BIOLOGY
IN THE POST GENOMIC ERA

BIOCOMPOSITES IN BIO-MEDICINE

MUDASIR AHMAD
MOHMMAD YOUNUS WANI
PREETI SINGH
SAIQA IKRAM
AND
BAOLIANG ZHANG
EDITORS

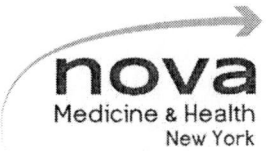

Copyright © 2019 by Nova Science Publishers, Inc.

All rights reserved. No part of this book may be reproduced, stored in a retrieval system or transmitted in any form or by any means: electronic, electrostatic, magnetic, tape, mechanical photocopying, recording or otherwise without the written permission of the Publisher.

We have partnered with the Copyright Clearance Center to make it easy for you to obtain permission to reuse content from this publication. Simply navigate to this publication's page on Nova's website and locate the "Get Permission" button below the title description. This button is linked directly to the title's permission page on copyright.com. Alternatively, you can visit copyright.com and search by title, ISBN, or ISSN.

For further questions about using the service on copyright.com, please contact:
Copyright Clearance Center
Phone: +1-(978) 750-8400   Fax: +1-(978) 750-4470   E-mail: info@copyright.com

NOTICE TO THE READER

The Publisher has taken reasonable care in the preparation of this book but makes no expressed or implied warranty of any kind and assumes no responsibility for any errors or omissions. No liability is assumed for incidental or consequential damages in connection with or arising out of the information contained in this book. The Publisher shall not be liable for any special, consequential, or exemplary damages resulting, in whole or in part, from the readers' use of, or reliance upon, this material. Any parts of this book based on government reports are so indicated and copyright is claimed for those parts to the extent applicable to compilations of such works.

Independent verification should be sought for any data, advice or recommendations contained in this book. In addition, no responsibility is assumed by the Publisher for any injury and/or damage to persons or property arising from any methods, products, instructions, ideas or otherwise contained in this publication.

This publication is designed to provide accurate and authoritative information with regard to the subject matter covered herein. It is sold with the clear understanding that the publisher is not engaged in rendering legal or any other professional services. If legal or any other expert assistance is required, the services of a competent person should be sought. FROM A DECLARATION OF PARTICIPANTS JOINTLY ADOPTED BY A COMMITTEE OF THE AMERICAN BAR ASSOCIATION AND A COMMITTEE OF PUBLISHERS.

Additional color graphics may be available in the e-book version of this book.

Library of Congress Cataloging-in-Publication Data

ISBN: 978-1-53616-247-9
Library of Congress Control Number:2019950487

Published by Nova Science Publishers, Inc. † New York

CONTENTS

Preface		vii
Chapter 1	Enzymatic Modification of Biopolymeric Surfaces for CO_2 Sequestration *Shalu Aggarwal, Arshiya Abbasi, Divyanshi Mangla, Suhail Ahmad, Kaiser Manzoor and Saiqa Ikram*	1
Chapter 2	Cellulose Based Nanocomposites for Biomedical and Pharmaceutical Applications *Sapana Jadoun*	29
Chapter 3	Application of Gelatin in Biomedical Field *Shikha Gupta*	49
Chapter 4	Polylactide (PLA) Based Nanocomposites for Applications in Antibacterial/Microbial and Biomedical Engineering *Sapana Jadoun*	69
Chapter 5	Polysaccharides Based Nanocomposites for Drug Delivery System *Anurakshee Verma*	87

Chapter 6	Polyvinyl Alcohol (PVA) Based Nanocomposites for Biomedical and Tissue Engineering Applications *Sapana Jadoun and Nirmala Kumari Jangid*	111
Chapter 7	Biopolymers and Their Role in Biomedicine *Javeed A Ganaie, Mudasir Ahmad and Baoliang Zhang*	127
Chapter 8	Lignin: A Wonderful Biopolymer *Bilal A. Bhat and Gulzar Rafiqi*	135
About the Editors		157
Index		163
Related Nova Publications		167

PREFACE

Biocomposites are a classic types of materials obtained from a matrix (renewable and non-renewable resources) and reinforcement of natural fibers. It often resembles the compositions of a living material implicated with a definite biological process. Industrialists and researcher's interest in biocomposites is rapidly growing due to the great benefits they offer such as being renewable, cheap, recyclable and biodegradable. The high potential for exploiting natural biopolymers with their broad range of structural, functional and physicochemical properties in various applications has provided the stimulus for the search for new or modified biocomposites. At present, research and development efforts in this field are relatively small, but the growing use of biocomposites based materials in wound healing management, drug delivery, and orthopedics repair products has stimulated scientists, engineers, and government agencies to put more efforts in fostering greater collaboration and bringing more advanced biopolymer-based biocomposites to replace the synthetically derived materials in biomedical applications.

The book covers the advanced traces of Biopolymers such as lignin, cellulose-based nanocomposites for biomedical and pharmaceutical applications, gelatin, polysaccharides based nanocomposites for applications in antibacterial/microbial/biomedical engineering, drug delivery system and tissue engineering. Further, presents the opportunities and applications in the field of biocomposites highlighting recent advances in areas commencing chemical synthesis and biosynthesis for end-user applications. This book will serve as a comprehensive literature guide for beginner researchers to grab the attention of biomedical researchers in both academia and industries to help streamline the efforts and understand the need to develop new biocomposites that could solve some of the most serious biomedical problems. The book is aimed to be a reference material for the academic and research community involved in biomedical research.

Finally, it is expected that this book will find a prominent place in the traditional universities and research institutions libraries where chemistry, biology technology, medicines as well as environmental studies, and other practical and theoretical mechanized topics are taught, studied and implemented.

In: Biocomposites in Bio-Medicine
Editors: Mudasir Ahmad et al.

ISBN: 978-1-53616-247-9
© 2019 Nova Science Publishers, Inc.

Chapter 1

ENZYMATIC MODIFICATION OF BIOPOLYMERIC SURFACES FOR CO_2 SEQUESTRATION

Shalu Aggarwal, Arshiya Abbasi, Divyanshi Mangla, Suhail Ahmad, Kaiser Manzoor, and Saiqa Ikram[*]

Bio/Polymers Research Laboratory, Department of Chemistry,
Jamia Millia Islamia, New Delhi-110025

ABSTRACT

Due to the increased demand for energy, which underlies the projected increase in CO_2 emission, parallel to clearing of the forests which reduces the photosynthesis to CO_2 from atmosphere; resulting in the net increase of CO_2 concentrations higher than earlier. Carbon sequestration–capturing and storing carbon emitted from the global energy system – could be a major tool for reducing atmospheric CO_2 emissions. Over last decades, Biopolymers are considered as most encouraging and assuring materials for modification of their surfaces due to the presence of amino, hydroxyl, carboxyl, sulphydryl, etc. functional groups among the biopolymers which contributes possible interactions among pollutants and biopolymers. With growing concern of environmental sustainability and non-biodegradation

---

[*] Corresponding Author's Email: sikram@jmi.ac.in.

of plastic waste, the biopolymers are emerging as the tool for the selective applications for reducing the pollution. Biopolymers are behind many important inventions of the past several decades, like 3D printing. So-called "engineering plastics," used in applications ranging from automotive to construction to furniture, have superior properties and can even help solve environmental problems; where the sequestration of CO_2 is in line with among the most prominent treatments. The arrays of biopolymers have been attempted with high precession and selectivity of CO_2 by many researchers. A series of modified biopolymer surfaces have been synthesized, to investigate the interaction between them with CO_2. The present chapter investigates and provides comprehensive information about the latest innovations in the biopolymers based renewable resources, along with the immobilization of different enzymes onto their surfaces to achieve the bio-mimicking for the above purpose.

Keywords: biopolymers, composite carriers, enzymes, modification of polymers, immobilization methods, applications

1. INTRODUCTION

From the earliest times, since life began Polymers have existed in natural forms such as DNA, RNA, proteins, and polysaccharides which play essential roles in plant and animal life. They are also known as macromolecules that are crucial to our very existence without which life seems very difficult. Large no. of single structural units called monomers are linked together in a regular manner by the chemical reaction known as polymerization give rise to the gaint molecule called "polymer". To form a molecule of high molecular weight, a chemical reaction occurs in which two or more substances coupled with or without an evolution of heat, water or any other solvents. With the growing advancements in the scientific and technological world, polymer chemistry plays an interesting role in providing solutions to the critical problems of food, cloth, shelter, education, air, health, energy resources, etc. As polymers serve comfort zone in the areas of medication, nutrition, communication, transportation, irrigation, recording history, buildings, etc.

In today's environment, renewability, recyclability, sustainability, triggered biodegradability all can make a huge difference. Eco-friendly composites, bio-composites derived from natural renewable resources having recycling capability and stability in their intended lifetime are called sustainable bio-based products. Cellulose, soy plastics, Microbial synthesized biopolymers i.e., polyhydroxyalkanoates (PHAs) polymers, starch is all the best-suited examples of biopolymers based on renewable resources.

Due to the presence of most preferable features in biomaterials such as molecular weight, material chemistry, shape and structure, solubility, lubricity, hydrophobicity, erosion mechanism, etc. they are perfectly considered for biomedical applications, tissue engineering scaffolds, and organ substitution. These materials improve the cell's performance in biological system since they exhibit bioactive properties and have better interactions with the cells. Numerous advantages are available for biodegradable polymeric materials over synthetic ones because of their versatile nature and have capability to not to accumulate or harm the environment. Some enlighten merits are the presence of important functional groups like amino, hydroxyl, Carboxyl on the surface of natural polymers which bear potential for tissue engineering and also less prone to produce toxic effects in the environment. Naturally, derived materials are biocompatible in nature and can be easily incorporated while synthetic ones are less compatible and get easily degraded into bio-products.

With the growing recent advances in biotechnology, various methods are employed for modification of biopolymer surfaces to achieve desired functional properties in such a way we are able to functionalize the surface of biopolymer by introducing some enviable functional groups so that it would be easy for biomacromolecules to interact with the surface of polymers. In this article, we are trying to familiarize the impact of recent advances in biotechnology as well as contemporary sciences of microbiology and interface between biotechnology and enzymology(S. Roller and 1. C. M. Dea. 1992). Before throwing the light on the impacts of biotechnology i.e., modification of biopolymers, the primary requirement is to figure out the concepts and the basic knowledge of biopolymers.

2. BIOPOLYMERS AS SUSTAINABLE RESOURCES

Biopolymers are acquired from plant and animal materials which can be grown indefinitely can be considered sustainable, and are always renewable. They are the guiding fundamentals for the polymers of next-generation which have nil impact, sustainability, eco-efficiency, and green chemistry. Over the last two decades, polymer chemistry has attracted the huge attention due to the extrusive or eye-catching apprehensions predominantly concern for the environment and secondly which is the major and most imperative reason i.e., recognition of synthetic materials or petroleum resources are finite that's why researchers nowadays fascinate towards the polymers which are renewable i.e., Biopolymers. The term "biopolymer" is also referred as organic polymer which is produced naturally by living organisms. Biodegradable or compostable polymeric materials can be derived from renewable resources under specific environmental conditions. One of the major blessings of biopolymer is that they are fully competent in biodegradation at accelerated rates, eco-friendly or used as green approaches by shattering down themselves into simple molecules such as carbon dioxide, methane or water by the action of microorganisms enzymatically in a limited period of time. Detailed classification of biopolymers on the basis of source or method of production given below:-

(i) Polymers such as polysaccharides or proteins which are directly extracted from biomass.
(ii) Polymers synthesized from renewable sources such as polylactic acid (PLA) by a classical chemical approach.
(iii) Polymers originated by genetical modification of bacteria such as polyhydroxyalkanoates (PHAs), bacterial cellulose, etc.

2.1. Natural Resources Derived from Fauna

2.1.1. Chitin and Chitosan

Chitin is the second most pervasive biopolymer present on the earth after cellulose (which comes under the category of fauna species and have discussed later in this chapter) and it is mainly found in the tightly bound complexes with other substances in the cuticles of crabs and shrimps as well as in the internal structure of invertebrates. It occurs in the forms of three allomorphs viz. α-Chitin, β-Chitin & γ-Chitin (a combination of both) which can merely individuated by infrared and solid-state NMR spectroscopies together. From the studies of these crystallographic invariants of two isomorphs, conclusion revealed that in α-Chitin, two antiparallel molecules per unit cell are present but only one parallel orientation exists in β-chitin, Islem Younes and Marguerite Rinaudo. (2015). The chains of α-Chitin & β-Chitin are organized in sheets and held by intra-sheet hydrogen bonds. Chitin is composed of β(1-4)-linked 2-acetamido-2-deoxy-β-D-glucose (N-acetylglucosamine) and often considered as cellulose derivative although it does not present in cellulose producing organisms but is structurally identical to cellulose despite it has acetamide groups (-NHCOCH$_3$) at the C-2 positions (Pradip Kumar Dutta et al. 2004). Chitin and its derivatives can be tailored or functionalized via certain chemical modifications like nitration, xanthation, sulphonation, acylation, phosphorylation, hydroxyalkylation, Schiff base formation, alkylation, ionic reactions or the one which is the most promising pathway of tailoring the chitin and its derivatives are graft polymerization. It is becoming a very optimistic remarkable material in this 21 century because of its advanced perspective on the grounds of medical, pharmaceutical, food industry, bio-science related advancements, tissue and protein engineering and so on (Keisuke Kurita 2006). Many researchers or authors have reviewed the laxation of chemical structure of chitin and chitosan in order to improve their solubility in conventional organic solvents (M. Jalal Zohuriaan-Mehr. 2005). Other biopolymers can easily blend or crosslinked with cell walls of many organisms and plants made up of chitin and can be cast into sheets or films. Because of having strong positive charge on the chitin and its derivatives, this property of natural biopolymer (chitin) can be exploited in many ways as we have seen its abundant applications in biomedical era. Due to its film-forming properties, it has enough potential for packaging materials in food packaging, edible films or coatings (Elisabeta Elena TĂNASE et al. 2014). This fascinating polymer has a huge variety of applications as well as chitosan which is a widely accepted biopolymer is extracted from chitin itself. On the other hand, Chitosan is a nitrogenous polysaccharide having amino group in its structural moiety called chitosan (poly-β-(1→4)-2-amino-2-deoxy-D-glucose) which is chiefly formed by deacetylation of chitin (George Z. Kyzas et al. 2015). Nowadays, Chitosan is becoming a very crucial topic especially in the fields of food, medical, protein or tissue engineering as well as in pharmaceutical applications. Chitosan is a marine polysaccharide that is widely used in biomedical research due to its encouraging properties like biocompatibility, biodegradability, low production cost, very little toxicity and highly abundant renewable material in the market. Its antibacterial activity has attracted wide attention to the researchers as this activity is affected by molecular weight and degree of acetylation where low molecular weight chitosan is harmless to the human body and has strong antimicrobial properties (Elisabeta Elena TĂNASE et al. 2014). Numerous natural polysaccharides of acidic in nature like cellulose, pectin, dextrin, alginic acid, agar, agarose are widely accepted or known to the researchers, among them, chitin and chitosan are the ones which are known for their basic nature due to the presence of amino groups which would be highly beneficial for chemical modifications. Now, moving towards to describe its preparation and its structural properties as chitosan is derived from deacetylation of α-chitin by giving aqueous alkali treatment i.e., 40 -50% at 120-150°C under heterogeneous conditions (Keisuke Kurita. 2006). This natural renewable polymer also is known as the deacetylated form of chitin. By repeated treatment of alkali, complete deacetylation of chitin can be achieved. The N-deacetylation of chitin can be implemented by homogeneously and heterogeneously approaches. Among these two, heterogeneous method can be considered best as it provides better results i.e., deacetylated up to 85-99% where homogeneous up to 45-55%. In heterogeneous method, chitin is treated with the hot concentrated solution of alkali NaOH during few hours which produced insoluble residue of chitosan. While in a homogeneous medium, chitin is dispersed in concentrated NaOH at 25°C for 3 hours or more than that, followed by dissolution in crushed ice around 0°C. This technique leads to the soluble chitosan with an average degree of acetylation of 48% - 55%. In nature, two types of chitin are available α-chitin and β-chitin. From these two types β-chitin from squid pens are most responsive to deacetylation reaction because of comparatively weak intermolecular forces of attraction, in addition to this, it tends to produce chitosan in a light tan to brown color under similar conditions (Keisuke Kurita. 2006). By deacetylation of chitin (poly-β-(1→4)-N-acetyl-D-glucosamine) which is one of the most interesting natural biopolymers, is mainly found in marine media and specifically in the exoskeleton of crustaceans or cartilages of mollusks, cuticles of insects and cell wall of microorganisms (George Z. Kyzas et al. 2015). Due to the availability of primary amino and secondary hydroxyl group, it is easily derivatized by introducing several functional groups which are easily accessible for interaction with the enzyme. To scrutinize their full potential, special stress has been put on structural metamorphosis of chitin and chitosan (Keisuke Kurita. 2006). In further discussion, the tailoring pathways for the modification of chitosan as renewable resources are explained.

Figure 1. Chemical Structure of chitin and chitosan.

2.1.2. Collagen

Special attention should also be paid to *collagen*. As collagen proteins are chiefly found in extracellular matrices of vertebrate animals. Being a natural polymer, collagen is a major structural component of tendon, bone and connective tissues of animal hides and skins that provides mechanical support and structural organization of connective tissues. Due to its biodegradable and biocompatible nature, collagen has outstanding applications in the field of biomedical grounds like tissue engineering, wound healing, drug delivery, and cosmetics. Moreover, for the improvement of the wound healing process, human tissues are replaced by animal-derived tissues because of the presence of collagen. It comprised of three polypeptide chains of triple helix and supramolecular structures are formed by all the members of the collagen family in extracellular matrix despite their variation in size, function and in tissue distribution (Figure 2) (K. Gelse et al. 2003). Collagen has been practiced for immobilization of tannase introducing glutaraldehyde as a cross-linking agent. Magnificent supporting matrix, Fe^{3+} collagen fibers have been proved beneficial for catalase immobilization as enzyme retains its significant activity even after 26 reuses (Sumitra Datta et al. 2012).

2.1.3. Alginates

Alginate is another natural polymer extracted from seaweeds that has gained tremendous interest in immobilization and microencapsulation technologies. It comprised of chains of alternating of α-L-guluronic acid and β-D-mannuronic acid residues (Figure 3). Carrier matrix of alginates is customarily built by crosslinking the carboxyl groups of α-L-guluronic acid with a solution of a cationic crosslinker such as barium chloride, calcium chloride and poly(L-lysine). Instability in the physiological environment or in the common buffer solutions with high concentration of phosphate and citrate ions that have ability to extract Ca^{2+} from the alginate matrices which are crosslinked with Ca^{2+} ions and liquefy the system is the major limitation of alginate matrices. In order to conquer the limitations of alginate as an immobilization material, numerous researchers or investigators have proposed to form microcapsule system or gel for protein immobilization by ionic complexation of chitosan (a positively charged material) and alginate (a negatively charged material). Several studies reveal that novel core-shell microcapsule technology for enzyme immobilization is proved to be very impressive technique in which enzyme is localized and protected in a core matrix, while the shell can regulate entry and exit of substrate and product. Chitosan crosslinked with sodium tripolyphosphate resulted in the phosphate ions diffusing into the Ca^{2+} alginate core and liquify it. Hence, we are in a condition to immobilize β-galactosidase in Ca^{2+} alginate (liquid core) as well as in Ba^{2+} alginate (solid core) enveloped by the perm-selective chitosan shell (Ehab Taqieddin et al. 2003). One of the major disadvantages is the leaching of enzyme from the support matrix of alginate when used without combination of any divalent ions such as Ca^{2+} ions or without any crosslinker like glutaraldehyde. To boost the interactions between enzyme and support matrix, composite of chitosan and alginate proved to be more reliable with high porosity and good hydrophilicity for trapping of enzyme (Sumitra Datta et al. 2012). This may be attributed to the presence of both hydroxyl & amino groups present in structure for covalent binding of enzyme.

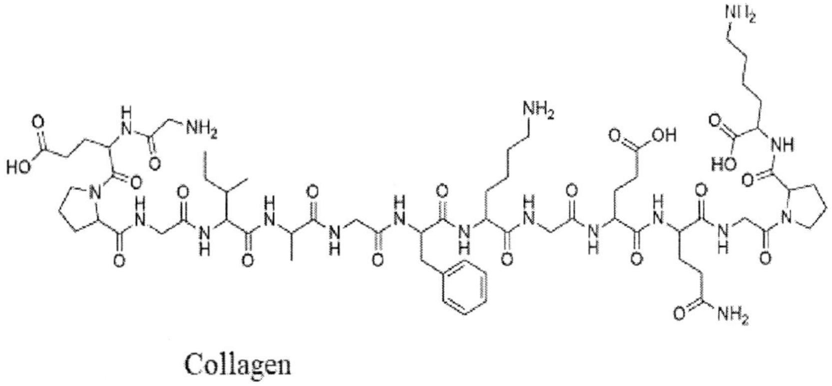

Figure 2. Chemical structure of collagen.

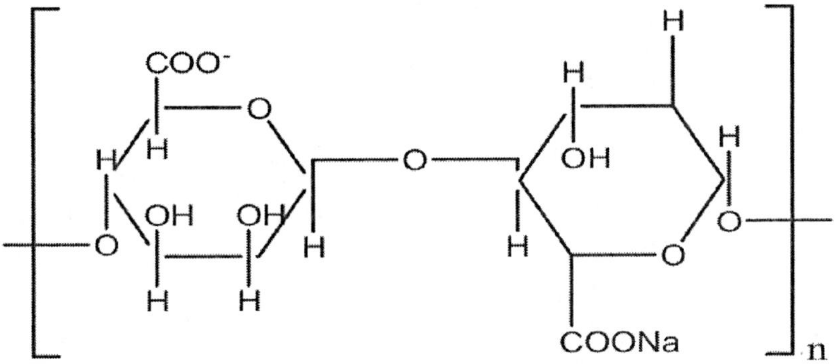

Figure 3. Chemical structure of alginate.

2.1.4. Gelatin

Gelatin is another renewable resource derived from natural resources like collagen taken from animal body parts which consist of many glycine residues, proline, and 4-hydroxy proline residues. The arrangement of the structure is Ala-Gly-Pro-Arg-Gly-Glu-4Hyp-Gly-Pro (Figure 4). It is most abundant polymer found in nature, possesses high hydrophilicity resulting in high swelling properties in aqueous media which helps in stabilizing in immobilizing the enzyme. It attracts attention for its use as a carrier matrix for an immobilized enzyme because it can be easily transformed into porous microcapsules. Earlier research papers revealed that gelatin would be used as a support matrix for the immobilization of glucoamylase (Exo-1,4-a-D-glucosidase) by cross-linking with glutaraldehyde followed by entrapment methodologies for the commercial process(J. F. Kennedy et al. 1984).

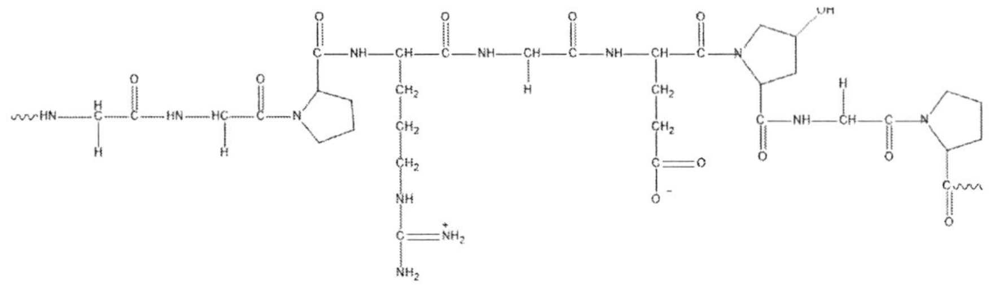

Figure 4. Chemical structure of gelatin.

2.2. Natural Resources Derived from Flora

2.2.1. Starch

Another striking and appreciating feature of biodegradable polymer is *Starch*. Due to its huge abundancy, cheaper and renewability, starch can minimize the use of synthetic polymers in plastic industries. Amylose and Amylopectin are the two main primary constituents of the starch. Although pure starch lacks mechanical strength despite this, it has been widely used in making biodegradable plastics (Elisabeta Elena TĂNASE et al. 2014). The hydrophilic nature of starch is the main limitation that inhibits its use in moisture environment. Entrapment of bitter-gourd peroxidase and surface immobilization of enzymes was carried out by calcium alginate-starch hybrid supports. In the presence of denaturants like urea entrapped enzyme was more stable due to internal carbohydrate moieties. In order to obtain high yield of products, industrial techniques are widely accepted such as grafting of substances like acrylamide & dimethylaminoethyl methacrylate on to starch for the immobilization process (Sumitra Datta et al. 2012).

2.2.2. Cellulose

Another very important and interesting biopolymer falls under the light of renewable resources which is known as unlimited and sustainable natural polymeric raw material having wide applications in grounds of both industries and domestic purposes. This raw material is mainly present in the form of microfibrils with the helical organization on the various levels containing domains of amorphous and crystallinity appearances. It is chiefly found in the cell walls of superior plants (Elisabeta Elena TĂNASE et al. 2014). The structure of cellulose reveals that it consists of linear chains of homopolysaccharide comprised of β-D-glucopyranose units linked together by β-1-4-linkages with a degree of polymerization (DP) of approximately 15000 for native cellulose cotton and 10000 for cellulose chain (Figure 6 represents the chemical structure of Cellulose unit). Mostly natural resources are characterized as rigid and partially crystalline materials. Cellulose is considered as the main constituent of compounds present on the earth especially within wood and natural fibers such as kenaf, palm, hemp, flax, etc. It lacks solubility in water, this property of cellulose reveals that it comprised of strong inter and intramolecular hydrogen bonding within and among individual chains. Consequently, the exterior surface of the cellulose fibers exhibits hydrophobic nature which renders it an assuring material for enzyme immobilization. Moreover, presence of hydroxyl groups on the cellulose surface proves to be an ideal site for taking part in covalent bonding of enzyme immobilization and also capable of bringing almost all the chemical reactions. The stability of cellulose is due to the formation of well-ordered hydrogen bonds because of the presence of hydroxyl groups on its surface of moiety of each monomer unit which is also a special evident in the crystalline packing of cellulose (Safwan Sulaiman et al. 2014).

Carboxymethylcellulose (CMC), cellulose acetate (CA) and cellulose nitrate are the few known derivatives of cellulose which are used as a raw material in chemical and biological industries at a high commercial level due to their features like inexpensive, non-toxic, biodegradable, and biocompatible (Yue Liu and Jonathan Y Chen. 2014).

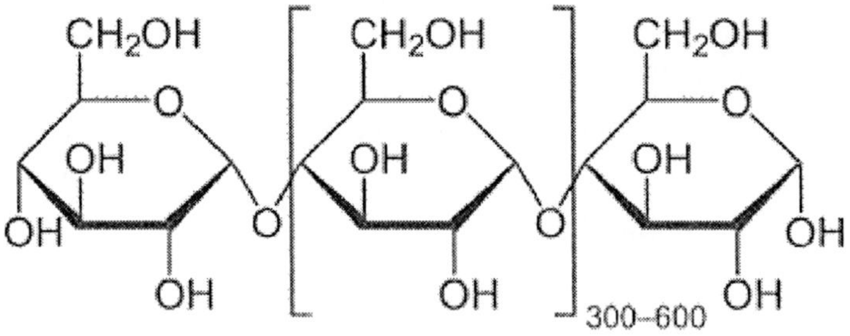

Figure 5. Chemical structure of starch.

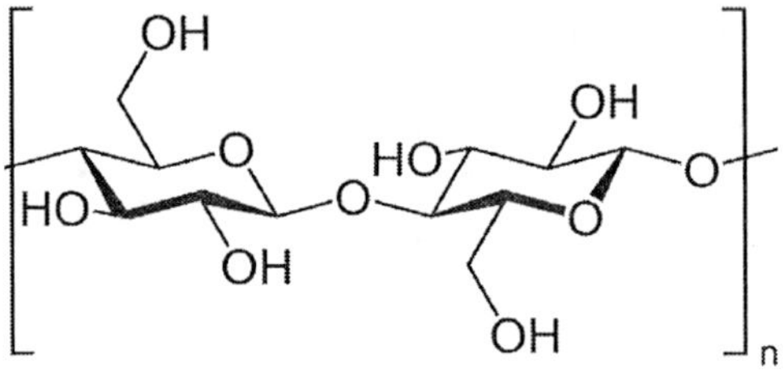

Figure 6. Chemical structure of cellulose unit.

2.2.3. Agar-Agar and Agarose

Agarose is one of the attractive biopolymer practiced in enzyme immobilization. Agar composed of two main components i.e., Agarose which is a linear neutral gelling heteropolysaccharide and Agaropectin is a heterogeneous mixture of smaller molecules. A major fraction of Agar i.e., agarose, a linear polymer consisting of two monosaccharide units i.e., (β-D-galactose) and (3,6-anhydrous-α-L-galactose) linked by glycosidic bonds β(1-4) & α(1-3) linkages. There are two repeating disaccharide units present in Agarose i.e., Agarobiose & neoagarobiose. Figure 7 represents the chemical structure of Agar-Agar & Agarose. 2 or 6 positions of 3,6-anhydrous-α-L-galactose residues can be substituted by $-OSO_3^-$,$-OCH_3$, glucuronate or pyruvate residues. Because of the presence of favorable functional properties, both agar and agarose gels have been used as a carrier matrix for electrophoresis and protein immobilization. Highly ordered stable and rigid structures can result without addition of any ions into the agarose solution at the temperature below 35°C which described its superlative ability of gelation (Jakub Zdarta et al. 2018). The most tempting feature of agar and agarose is their ability to form stable and firm gels. Moreover, agarose is an extremely inert colloid and possesses an outstanding strong hydrophilic and lyophilic nature in aqueous solutions that provides an ideal site for enzyme immobilization (Paolo Zucca et al. 2016).

In addition to inertness and stiffness, beads based on agarose are highly porous, mechanically resistant, chemically and physically inert and sharply hydrophilic. Linear galactan polysaccharide agar belongs to the Rhodophyceae class and is extracted from seaweeds. Agar/Agarose gels are suitably advised for immobilization because having ability to form derivatives as each monomer agarobiose unit has four alcoholic functional groups in which three of them are secondary and one is primary functional group that is the main target of derivatizations. Though 100% derivation is neither accessible nor commendable, few chemical reagents such as amine, carboxyl, sulfonate, cyano and so on can be grafted along with the polymer chain. For example, Glyoxal agarose in which the primary hydroxyl group is etherified by glycidol to produce diols which further oxidized by sodium periodate to get glyoxal group has been proved an excellent covalent attachment with an enzyme.

2.3. Inorganic Composite Carriers

Inorganic matrixes are prudently contemplated for enzyme immobilization because of superlative features such as the highest degree of thermal and mechanical resistance, rigidity, porosity moreover these supports are completely resistant for bacterial and fungal growth. A comprehensive discussion about the properties of inorganic supports is beyond the capacity of this chapter, therefore, we are presenting only some miscellaneous features of inorganic carriers for enzyme immobilization.

2.3.1. Silica-Based Supports

Silicon dioxide (SiO_2) exists as a 3-D polymer in which SiO_4 tetrahedra units are arranged by sharing their vertices and composed a rigid entity while the Si-O-Si angles are highly flexible which shows remarkable polymorphs of silica ranging from highly ordered crystalline forms to mesoporous amorphous solids. Quartz and cristobalite are the crystalline forms of SiO_2. Natural mineral viz. stishovite is another metastable form of SiO_2 obtained by applying high temperature and pressure conditions on silica solids where each silicon atom is hosted within an octahedral cluster of six oxygen atoms such as it appears as a rutile form of titania (TiO_2) is extremely compact and unreactive towards mineral acids. Silica-based materials have combination of both hydrophobic and hydrophilic sites on its surface having a high tendency to show hydrogen bonding which describes complex adsorptive properties of immobilizing enzymes onto the surface of silica. Glutaraldehyde or 3-aminopropyltriethoxysilane is the surface modifying agents that facilitate the enzyme attachment with the hydroxyl groups present on its surface (Paolo Zucca and Enrico Sanjust. 2014). Various enzymes like oxidoreductases, transferases, hydrolases or isomerases have been immobilized on sol-gel silica, fumed silica, colloidal silica nanoparticles with high catalytic retention and good thermal or mechanical properties. (Jakub Zdarta et al. 2018).

2.3.2. Ceramics

The phrase '*ceramics*' chiefly illustrates metal oxides or mixed metallic/non-metallic oxides based on inorganic and non-metallic materials. These materials are suitable for immobilizing proteins because of encouraging properties such as they exhibit extremely high resistance to temperature, pressure, and chemicals and also provide the highest degree of mechanical strength. The unique feature of these materials is when enzymes become catalytically inactive, they get easily regenerated and again used for the immobilization of new biocatalyst. Non-specific interactions are possible due to the presence of hydroxyl groups on their surface which facilitates adsorption immobilization of enzymes. Alumina, Titania, Zirconia, Iron-oxide, Silica, and Calcium phosphate, Composite ceramic membranes (TiO_2/Al_2O_3) are several ceramic materials which have been used as a biomolecule carrier for immobilizing enzymes (Jakub Zdarta et al. 2018).

2.3.3. Alumina

Corundum being abundant in nature called Alumina i.e., Aluminium oxide (Al_2O_3) obtained from aluminum ores in hydrated form. Different crystalline forms of alumina could be prepared either by strong heating of Aluminium hydroxide ($Al(OH)_3$) or by applying the base treatment on aqueous aluminum salts. All these forms appear to have high porosity, high specific surface but can change into α-Alumina on heating above 1000°C which shows inert nature and devoid of any interest in the field of protein immobilization. Other crystalline forms (η & γ-Alumina) are obtained by moderate calculations called sandy alumina which could represent alternatives for silica-based supports. The surfaces of this alumina are coordinatively unsaturated and this feature is responsible for both catalytic and adsorptive properties and can seldom found as a support for enzyme immobilization (Paolo Zucca and Enrico Sanjust. 2014).

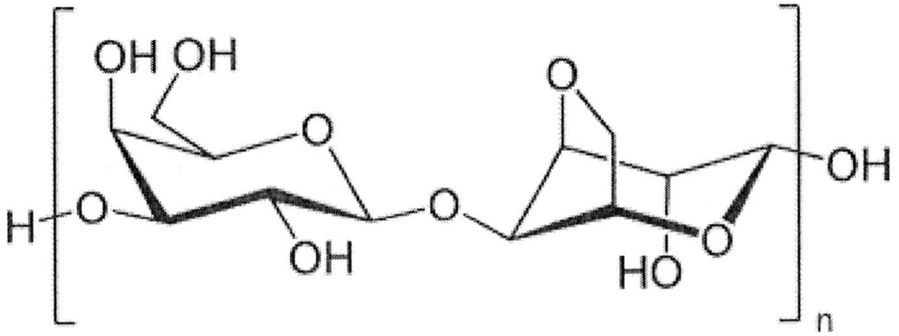

Figure 7. Chemical structure of agar-agar and agarose.

2.3.4. Carbon-Based Materials

During the last two decades, activated carbons, modified and unmodified charcoals are some prototypes of Carbon-based materials have been used as effective and valuable support materials in enzyme immobilization. The promising features of these materials are a presence of various functional groups, high adsorption capacity, well-developed porous structure having various sizes and volumes, high surface area (up to 1000 m^2/g), the minimal release of fine particulate matters make carbon-based materials suitable carriers for the adsorption immobilization of various enzymes. For instance, amyloglucosidase was immobilized on unmodified charcoal support.

2.4. Classic Materials

Both inorganic and Organic materials are termed as Classic materials used for enzyme immobilization have been described in the above sections. Silica-based supports, carbon-based materials, inorganic oxides, ceramics which have described under the category of Inorganic and Composite carriers are acknowledged for their good sorption properties, thermal and chemical stability as well as by excellent mechanical resistance. All these astonishing features ensure numerous contact sites for effective enzyme immobilization. Auxiliary materials such as biopolymers and synthetic polymers also assembled under classic materials endeavors various functional groups which facilitates even covalent binding of enzymes without cross-linking agents. With respect to synthetic polymers, biopolymers are consistently symbolized by high protein affinity as well as biocompatibility that restraint negative effects of the support on the structure of enzymes. Moreover, Classic materials are found lavishly in nature (mineral, biopolymers) and are effortlessly synthesize which makes them relatively cheap. These superlative facts of these materials play an imperative role as carriers for use for the immobilization of enzymes. Summarized form of Classic materials and types of enzymes that may be immobilized using these supports grouped with information about immobilization type, cross-linking agents and binding group in tabular form is given below (Jakub Zdarta et al. 2018) (Table 1).

Table 1. Summary and selected examples of Classic materials of both inorganic and organic origin applied for enzymes immobilization

Support Material	Binding groups	Crosslinking Agents	Immobilization Type	Immobilized Enzyme
Inorganic Materials				
Activated Charcoal	-OH, C=O, COOH	-	Adsorption	Papain
Sol-gel Silica	-OH	-	Adsorption	Lipase from *Aspergillusniger*
Silica gel	-OH, C=O	glutaraldehyde	Covalent Binding	Commercial lipase
Commercial Activated Carbon	-OH, C=O	-	Adsorption	Cellulose from *Aspergillus niger*
Organic Materials				
Polyaniline	$-NH_2$, C=O	Glutaraldehyde	Covalent Binding	α-amylase
Polyvinyl alcohol	-OH, C=O	Glutaraldehyde	Covalent Binding	Laccase from *Trametes Versicolor*
Polystyrene	C=O, epoxy groups	Poly(glycidyl methacrylate)	Covalent Binding	lipase
Chitosan	-OH, $-NH_2$	Glutaraldehyde	Entrapment	Lipase from *Candida rugosa*
Agarose	-OH	-	Entrapment	α-amylase
Cellulose nanocrystals	-OH	-	Adsorption	Lipase from *Candida rugosa*

3. IMPACT MODIFICATION OF ENGINEERING BIOPOLYMERIC SURFACES AND BULKS

The unique proposition or the main agenda of this chapter is to bring out various modifications or functionalization of the surfaces of biopolymers and introduce some new functionality. Over the last few decades, researchers have focussed on the investigation and utilization of microbial cellulose in functional materials. Functional bacterial cellulose-based materials are enough capable to produce improved or new properties by mixing multiple constituents and exploiting synergistic effects such as electronic, optical, magnetic and catalytic properties. The performance of biopolymers must be increased in order to extend its applications in immobilizing the proteins or other macromolecules. Alterations or fabrications are done by incorporation of fillers and reinforcements, blending, plasticization & impact modifications. The development of novel polymeric materials is the fastest method in tailoring the properties of polymers which consequently play a very crucial role in increasing the competitiveness and biocompatibility of biopolymers. Figure 8 describes all the possible techniques of surface modification.

3.1. Physically Modified Biopolymers

3.1.1. Biopolymer Composites

Biocomposites are the modified form of biopolymers which can be made by incorporation of fillers and reinforcements into a polymer matrix results in a heterogeneous system. Comprehensive work done by several researchers stated that under the effect of external load heterogeneities induce stress concentration, the magnitude of which depends on the geometry of the inclusions, on the elastic properties of the components and on interfacial adhesion. Overall performance of the composites, deformation and failed behavior is determined by heterogeneous stress distribution and local stress maximums initiate local micromechanical deformations. Another factor that must be taken into account during the analysis of micromechanical deformation processes is the interaction of the components. Characters and strength both factors are present in interactions. Secondary forces created by adhesive interactions are relatively weak. The coupling may result in covalent bonding between the components.

Most studies focus on the potential use of natural lignocellulose fibers i.e., wood flour, sisal, flax, etc. for modification of biopolymers. Biocomposite materials have wide applications in the building and automotive industry. Renewable and biodegradable based matrices are the leading carriers due to growing environmental concerns. PLA (polylactic acid) is one of the most important biopolymers which is frequently used for the production of fiber-reinforced composites.

Biocomposites are present in nanometre-scale called bio-nano composites possessing unique characteristics with respect to gas and water vapor permeability, thermal stability, fire resistance, mechanical and optical properties, etc. Alternatively, these characteristics can be modified using either natural nanofibers such as cellulose or inorganic nanofillers such as silica, layered silicates, etc. different combinations of properties are achieved. In order to achieve nanoscale dispersion, i.e., intercalated or exfoliated structure resulting in superior properties, nano clays must be modified with suitable organic compounds in order to promote the separation of the silicate layers (Paolo Zucca et al. 2016).

3.1.2. Blends

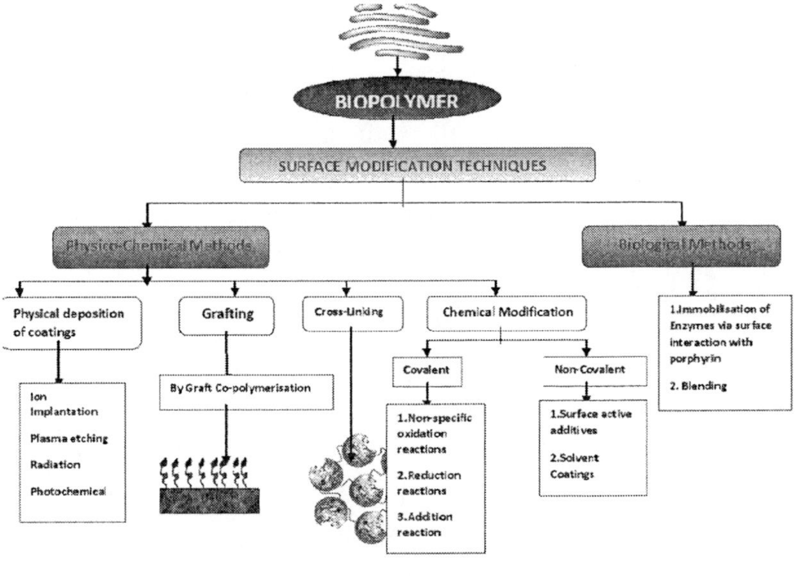

Figure 8. Surface modification techniques.

By Physical blending, we figure out that in fused state polymeric materials are simply fused or blend without causing any chemical reaction to occur. To create new materials with desired combination of properties, this is a satisfactory route. In this process, no extra investment is required and this process can be carried out by using conventional machinery which is a crucial aspect for industry. With the help of this technique, we can target our application in a very short interval of time and at cheaper rates as compared to the development of new monomers and polymerization techniques. Polylactic acid (PLA), starch is the most often used material for physical blending process.

3.2. Chemically Modified Biopolymers

Another major approach for immobilization of macromolecules on the biopolymeric surfaces is "Chemical modification". For this purpose, ample of chemical reactions and reagents have been explored. The procedure of surface tailoring begins with the surface activation, which creates desirable functionalities on the surface of polymer that enables the surface immobilization of ligands under mild conditions. Earlier, several methods have been proposed to create 3-D scaffolds of varying size, shape, and architecture, still are challenging situations. Alkali hydrolysis of aliphatic polyester surfaces is the most frequently used technique in chemical modification method. As alkali treatment is driven by small, highly mobile protons that can diffuse easily between the uncharged polymer chains and therefore has the capability to penetrate into porous 3-D scaffolds. New active functionalities are created after surface hydrolysis that causes the cleavage of ester bonds, which results in the formation of free hydrophilic carboxyl and hydroxyl functionalities that permits the covalent attachment of other biomolecules such as enzymes or proteins on the surface of the polymer. Mostly, ligands have a biological origin for improving cell interactions. After hydrolysis, biodegradable polymers like PLA (polylactic acid), PLGA (poly lactic-co-glycolic acid) undergo conjugation with primary amines are mostly accepted. Common diamines which are used in this procedure are ethylenediamine,1,6-hexane diamine, N-aminoethyl-1,3-propane diamine, etc. For instance, carboxylate groups can also be activated by the formation of a highly active species which are generated by carbodiimides after further reactions with amine nucleophiles that leads to the stable amide bonds. The most fascinating methodology is to introduce nitrogen and sulfur moieties with the help of N-hydroxysuccinimide (NHS) or N-hydroxysulfosuccinimide (Sulfo-NHS) to form stable ester derivatives. Signaling proteins can then be immobilized on aminolysis matrices/ scaffolds with the help of these cross-linking agents (Jakub Zdarta et al. 2018).

3.3. Plasma Treated

The surface properties of the biomaterials can be altered without affecting their bulk properties by technique called Plasma. To enable the creation of glow discharge plasma, low-pressure gases such as argon, ammonia or oxygen are filled in the evacuated vessel. Energy sources such as electric discharge, heat, radio-frequency energy, alternating/direct current are able to excite the gas. Free radicals, ions, protons, electrons, gas atoms and molecules of different energies are generated by ionization of gases. Successive bombardment with these high energy species on biopolymer surfaces results in the transfer of energy from plasma to the substrate which consequently leads to chemical and physical changes on the surface of the substrate. A very interesting feature of plasma technique that these energetic species can interact with polymer surface ranges from several hundred angstroms to 10 microns without inducing any changes in their bulk composition. Cold or low-temperature plasma & hot or elevated temperature plasma are the two major types of plasma where hot plasma is generated by atmospheric pressure arcs while low-temperature glow discharge generates cold plasma. From these two types, cold or low-temperature plasma is often preferred over hot plasma because, in high-temperature plasma, thermal motion of surface molecules is high and is very difficult to maintain whereas plasma generated effects in low plasma are efficiently maintained. Earlier studies have been acknowledged the use of plasma techniques for surface modification of polymers. By using plasma techniques in functionalization and alteration of polymeric surfaces, various studies came across numerous attractive and fascinating qualities such as enhanced cell adhesion, surface wettability, improved biocompatibility, and molecular immobilization.

Moreover, this can also lead to improving surface hydrophilicity of the polymer.

3.4. Photochemical Modification

Surfaces of biopolymers can be modified photochemically through free radical polymerization which results in polymer cross-linking, photopolymerization of monomers or grafting of molecules. Free radicals are generated by highly energetic UV rays, X-rays, γ-rays or by photo-initiators to initiate the chemical reactions on the surface of the biopolymers. Thus, radicals which are generated then interacts with another monomer molecule that ultimately leads to the propagation of the reaction and polymer chain formation. Organic compounds such as alkyl hydroperoxides (R-OOH) or halogens are some common photo-initiators required in these modifications. It is very beneficial technique with respect to other modifications due to selective immobilization of the target species at specific regions of the biomaterial, forming graft layers. Established studies adopt protocols of photo-polymerization for creating functionalities for applications of tissue engineering. This chapter reveals introduction of various functional groups such as (-OH), (-COOH), and (-CONH$_2$) to activate the surface of biopolymer by applying photo-grafting treatment on hydroxyethyl methacrylate, methacrylic acid or acrylamide respectively. Presently, there are two approaches by which immobilization of proteins was performed. In the first one surface of biomaterials such as collagen and gelatin can be activated by methyl sulphonyl chloride followed by adsorption of proteins. And in second one, polymer film can be activated via EDAC treatment followed by immersion in gelatin and collagen solution. Consequently, wettability of the surface was improved. For tissue engineering applications, numerous photopolymerization studies have been conducted on polymeric films and have produced astonishing results (Jakub Zdarta et al. 2018).

4. APPLICATIONS OF BIOPOLYMERS: GLOBAL SCENARIO

4.1. In Biotechnology

In the above sections, we have discussed physical adsorption, chemical modification, treatment through photochemically and via plasma methodology for protein immobilization. This portion briefly debates on protein immobilization having focus on the development of protein delivery systems as an approach towards tissue engineering. Numerous carrier matrix based on renewable biomaterials has been explored over the last two decades such as protein encapsulated hydrogels. Several published articles disclosed that although physical adsorption or entrapment/encapsulation are the leading methods for immobilization of proteins studies also revealed that bioactivity of enzymes is lost due to their random orientations, over-crowding and rapid desorption of adsorbed proteins or due to the short half-lives of signaling proteins combined with reduced bioavailability. For these reasons, protein delivery systems based on adsorption or entrapment are restraint. So, the concept of covalent immobilization of proteins is achieving higher heights for tissue engineering applications. This technique implements oriented immobilization with minimum structure losses, conformation and protein spreading. Minimum spreading permits immobilized protein to become more realistic and quantized. Moreover, immobilization through covalent binding diminishes the amount of signaling/therapeutic protein essential for provoking an appropriate function as compared to adsorption techniques. Protein can be readily used for covalent binding with polymeric surfaces due to the presence of a variety of functional groups such as amino groups, carboxyl groups, hydroxyl and thiol moieties on the surface of proteins.

4.2. For Enzyme Immobilisation

There are two approaches by which proteins can be covalently immobilized on biopolymeric surfaces i.e., (i) By tailoring the structures of proteins and polymers or (ii) By chemically crosslinking between protein and polymer surfaces. Random and oriented covalent attachments are the two broad categories of Covalent attachments.

Previous papers revealed that a known hormone called insulin was successfully immobilized onto the polymers with the help of water-soluble carbodiimides as a cross-linking agent that is capable to form a covalent bond between the carboxyl group of the polymer and the amine terminals on proteins.

Another approach is also implemented in industries known as Oriented covalent immobilization where protein activity is critical and has the ability to reuse immobilized protein multiple times. Several reagents and cross-linkers that have been used as degradable and non-degradable have published for specific modifications of protein and biomaterial attachment. Prognosis about polymer and protein attachment still remains a challenge because of extreme diversity, sensitivity, and complexity of signaling/ therapeutic proteins. Moreover, threat is consistently maintained for protein denaturation due to the use of chemicals and crosslinkers. Therefore, the urgent contribution is required for improving the performances that can overcome these limits (Jakub Zdarta et al. 2018, Paolo Zucca et al. 2016, Paolo Zucca et al. 2014).

4.3. For CO_2 Sequestration

In order to reduce the level of carbon dioxide released in the atmosphere, biomimetic sequestration of carbon dioxide is one of the proposed methods comes under the various studies. To alleviate the challenges of carbon dioxide, biodegradable, biocompatible and thermostable biopolymers such as (Polyhydroxyalkanoates (PHAs) are introduced into the system as they are capable of fixing atmospheric CO_2 into useful products like calcium carbonate ($CaCO_3$). Biopolymer such as chitosan contains large no. of amino functional groups which can be chemically modified to undergo intermolecular hydrogen bonding that facilitates the acidic CO_2 molecule to get adsorbed on to the surface of the polymer. CO_2 uptake capacity increases by crosslinking and functionalization of biopolymers.

Moreover, carbonic anhydrase enzyme which is mainly present in the red corpuscles in the human blood is capable of inter-conversion of CO_2 into harmless products; such as bicarbonates and hydrogen ions. Similarly, enzymatic systems are designed for sequestration or biomineralization of atmospheric CO_2 into solid carbonates or in the production of commodity fuels and chemicals.

CONCLUSION AND FUTURE ENDEAVOURS

Surface or bulk modifications of biopolymers via immobilizing or covalently attached proteins, carbohydrates, lipids, and any other species is incredibly important for several reasons. It is well known that a series of interactions occur between the surfaces of biopolymers and the chemical ligands after they have been implemented into a particular environment. Hence biopolymers surfaces are playing an extremely important role in the response towards artificial medical devices to the biological environment. To transform any surface, to be hydrophilic or hydrophobic, there are lots of possibilities. In the presented chapter, comprehensive literature is compiled for the functionalization of polymer surface properties via protein/peptide immobilization. In this compilation, the enzyme (carbonic anhydrase) has been given special attention in various researches for carbon dioxide sequestration. The performance of immobilized carbonic anhydrase has been greatly improved when it was immobilized on polyester polymer via covalent method. Furthermore, this article provides an insight into the development of the new natural polymer-based materials for environmental applications particularly in carbon dioxide capture and its biomineralization and biotransformation. To characterize the operating life span of both native carbonic anhydrase and the enzyme mimics particularly after immobilization, however, more work needs to be conducted and new elaborative research needs to be focused on the methods of immobilization that would immobilize enzyme especially carbonic anhydrase (CA) for CO_2 sequestration that will control Global warming to the larger extent.

REFERENCES

Elisabeta Elena, TĂNASE., Maria, RÂPĂ. & Ovidiu, POPA. (2014). "Biopolymers Based on Renewable Resources - A Review." *Scientific Bulletin. Series F. Biotechnologies*, *18*, 2285-1364.

Ehab Taqieddin. & Mansoor, Ameji. (2003). "Enzyme immobilization in novel alginate-chitosan core-shell microcapsules." *Biomaterials*, *25*, 1937-1945.

George, Z. Kyzasand. & Dimitrios, N. Bikiaris. (2015). "Recent Modifications of Chitosan for Adsorption Applications: A Critical and Systematic Review." *Mar. Drugs*, *13*, 312-337.

Gelse, K., poschl, E. & Aigner, T. (2003). "Collagens-structure, function and biosynthesis." *Advanced Drug Delivery Reviews*, *55*, 1531-1546.

Islem, Younes. & Marguerite, Rinaudo. (2015). "Chitin and Chitosan Preparation from Marine Sources. Structure, Properties and Applications." *Marine Drugs*, *13*, 1133-1174.

Jalal Zohuriaan-Mehr, M. (2005). "Advances in Chitin and Chitosan Modification through Graft Copolymerization: A Comprehensive Review." *Iranian Polymer Journal*, *14* (3), 235-265.

Jakub, Zdarta., Anne, S. Meyer., Teofil, Jesionowski. & Manuel, Pinelo. (2018). "A General Overview of Support Materials for Enzyme Immobilization: Characteristics, Properties, Practical Utility." *Catalysts*, *8*, 92; doi:10.3390/catal8020092.

Keisuke, Kurita. (2006). "Chitin and Chitosan: Functional Biopolymers from Marine Crustaceans." *Marine Biotechnology*, *8*, 203–226.

Kennedy, J. F. & Kalogerakisand, B. & Cabral, J. M. S. (1984). "Immobilization of enzymes on crosslinked gelatin particles activated with various forms and complexes of titanium (IV) species." *Enzyme Microb. Technol.*, *6*, 0141 –0229.

Pradip, Kumar Dutta., Joydeep, Dutta. & Tripathi, V. S. (2004). "Chitin and chitosan: Chemistry, properties and applications." *Journal of Scientific & Industrial Research*, *63*, 20-31.

Paolo, Zucca., Roberto, Fernandez-Lafuente. & Enrico, Sanjust. (2016). "Agarose and Its Derivatives as Supports for Enzyme Immobilization." *Molecules*, *21*, 1577; doi:10.3390/molecules21111577.

Paolo, Zucca. & Enrico Sanjust. (2014). "Inorganic Materials as Supports for Covalent Enzyme Immobilization: Methods and Mechanisms." *Molecules*, *19*, 14139-14194, doi:10.3390/molecules190914139.

Roller, S. & Dea, I. C. M. (1992). "Biotechnology in the Production and Modification of Biopolymers for Foods." *Critical Reviews in Biotechnology*, *12*(3), 261-277.

Sumitra, Datta., Rene Christena, L. & Yamuna, Rani Sriramulu Rajaram. (2012). "Enzyme immobilization: an overview on techniques and support materials." *Biotech*, (2013), 3, 1–9 DOI 10.1007/s13205-012-0071-7.

Safwan, Sulaiman., Mohd Noriznan, Mokhtar., Mohd Nazli Naim., Azhari, Samsu Baharuddin. & Alawi, Sulaiman. (2014). "A Review: Potential Usage of Cellulose Nanofibers (CNF) for Enzyme Immobilization via Covalent Interaction." *Applied Biochem Biotechnol*, (2015), *175*, 1817–1842.

Yue, Liu. & Jonathan, Y. Chen. (2014). "Enzyme immobilization on cellulose matrixes." *Journal of Bioactive and Compatible Polymers*, 1–15. DOI: 10.1177/0883911516637377.

In: Biocomposites in Bio-Medicine
Editors: Mudasir Ahmad et al.
ISBN: 978-1-53616-247-9
© 2019 Nova Science Publishers, Inc.

Chapter 2

CELLULOSE BASED NANOCOMPOSITES FOR BIOMEDICAL AND PHARMACEUTICAL APPLICATIONS

Sapana Jadoun[*]
School of Basic & Applied Sciences, Department of Chemistry,
Lingayas Vidyapeeth, Faridabad, Haryana, India

ABSTRACT

In recent years cellulose-based nanocomposites have gained attention owing to the enhanced mechanical, thermal, high strength and stiffness, renewability and biodegradability, along with their production and application in the expansion of composites. These are emerging renewable nanocomposites that hold potential in many different applications such as food, chemicals, personal care, packaging and products, automotive, construction, electronics and furniture along with. High-performance nanocomposites can be prepared by appropriate modification of cellulose fibers as reinforcement material, resulting in improved physical, chemical as well as biological properties. The chapter provides an overview of cellulose nanocomposites focusing on the processing, properties, and applications in pharmaceutical and biomedical fields.

---

[*] Corresponding Author's Email: sjadoun022@ gmail.com.

Keywords: cellulose, nanocomposites, pharmaceutical, biomedical

1. INTRODUCTION

Cellulose is the most plentiful form of living terrestrial biomass material in nature (Crawford 1981) which is a common plant biopolymer, complex polysaccharide or carbohydrate comprising of 3,000 or more glucose units with 33 percent of all vegetable matter and the annual production is estimated to be around 10^{11} tons. It is a natural polymer, which is a long chain macromolecule and made by the linkage of smaller molecules. In the cellulose chain, the links are made by consisting of sugar, β-D-glucose (Dorée 1947). These sugar units are connected when water is removed by merging the H and –OH group. Above two of these sugars linkage results, a disaccharide is known as cellobiose (Kalia et al. 2011). Cellulose is most profuse of all naturally existing organic compounds and it is the basic structural component of the cell wall. In 1980, *Anselm Payen* (Payen 1838) first recognized the existence of cellulose as the communal material of plant cell walls. Several natural fibers like cotton and higher plants have cellulose as their main component. It comprises of long chains of anhydrous-D-glucopyranose units (AGU) and is insoluble in water as well as most common solvents. Therefore, chemical modification of cellulose is performed to enhance processability and to yield cellulosic (cellulose derivatives) so that they can be tailored for specific industrial applications. Cellulose has been widely investigated due to its advantageous properties, like low-cost, hydrophilicity, non-toxicity, biocompatibility, biodegradeability, low density, combustible and nonabrasive (Fu et al. 2019).

Composites are a combination of two or more different components with knowingly different chemical and physical properties. They have improved mechanical performance along with new functionalities. Generally, a composite contains a stiff and strong component known as the reinforcement which is embedded in a softer constituent, the matrix. In this way, the composite has advantageous properties of reinforcement and the matrix. Composites can be classified into three categories in terms of matrix used are (1) ceramic matrix composites (2) metal matrix composites (3) polymer matrix composites. There are many thermoplastic polymers like poly (ethylene) (Lu, Lin, and Chen 2007), poly (ethylene oxide) (Chen and Tsubokawa 2000) and poly (vinyl chloride) (Chazeau et al. 1999) while thermosetting polymers like phenolic resin (Zárate, Aranguren, and Reboredo 2008), unsaturated polyester (Vilay et al. 2008), rubber (Setua and De 1984) and epoxy resin (Zhou et al. 2006). With increased awareness on environmental protection and sustainability, researchers have been shown interest in yield biodegradable polymer composites based on starch (Kvien et al. 2007) poly (lactic acid) (Bondeson and Oksman 2007) and cellulose (Gindl and Keckes 2005). Composites achieve the properties of both reinforcement and matrix with enhanced properties of compressive and strengths. Booker and Boysen (2005) presented special efforts towards nanotechnology and gave a high expectation for researchers. A nanoparticle is usually considered when as a minimum one of the linear dimensions is lesser than 100 nm (Henriksson et al. 2007). The perspective of nanocomposites in several areas of research and application is auspicious and attracting. Nanocomposite materials have many advantages properties like their superior mechanical, thermal, and barrier properties at low reinforcement levels along with their transparency, low weight, and better recyclability when compared with conventional composites (Oksman et al. 2006; Sorrentino, Gorrasi, and Vittoria 2007). Loads of research works have been carried out all over the world for the preparation of various types of nanocomposites by using cellulose fibers as a reinforcing material. The main reason to utilize cellulose nanofibers in composite materials is that one can potentially exploit the high stiffness of the cellulose crystal for reinforcement. This can be done by breaking down the hierarchical structure of the plant into individualized nanofibers of high crystallinity, with a reduction of amorphous parts.

2. METHODS

2.1. Cellulose Nanocomposite Processing

Processing of nanocomposites of cellulose makes them suitable candidate for low-cost engineering material with plant fiber reinforcement in industry (Berglund and Peijs 2010) along with its cheaper, renewable and low abrasive nature, impressive mechanical properties, abundance, low weight, and biodegradability of cellulose nanocrystals (Azizi Samir, Alloin, and Dufresne 2005; Oksman et al. 2002; Hornsby, Hinrichsen, and Tarverdi 1997; Bledzki, Reihmane, and Gassan 1996). In determining the composite properties, processing condition plays an important role such as Glass fibers have high strength when freshly drawn whereas the condition was altered i.e., exposed to humid air then fibers absorb water surfaces of fibers become damaged because of rubbing action during processing, the strength decreases. The temperature of processing is also restricted for specific materials like for lignocellulosic materials, it is controlled to about 200°C due to their degradation temperature starts from 230°C (Hamad 2013). Cellulose nanocomposites can be processed using conventional processing methods. Before processing, drying of fibers is the key point as the water content in the fiber can outcome in weak adhesion in between fiber and polymer or it may cause voids in the nanocomposite when the water evaporates during processing.

Nishino, Matsuda, and Hirao (2004) reported the two typical routes for the preparation of cellulose nanocomposites, one-step and two-step methods (Figure 1). In this method, cellulose is firstly dissolved in a solvent which was followed by regeneration of the cellulose in the existence of another cellulose component which was undissolved. Vallejos, Peresin, and Rojas (2012) synthesized all-cellulose composites by electrospinning cellulose acetate (CA) solution having dispersed cellulose nanocrystals (CNC) to yield precursor CA/CNC composites. However, in the one-step method, cellulosic fibers are slightly dissolved in a solvent and then redeveloped in situ to obtain a matrix around the undissolved part. Cellulose composites are prepared using different composites manufacturing techniques like injection molding, resin transfer molding (RTM), compression molding and vacuum bagging. Rånby (1951); Ranby (1952) firstly synthesized cellulose nanocrystals by hydrolysis of cellulosic biomass in mineral acid (hydrochloric or sulfuric). Processing starts with milling the pulp for small uniform particles followed by acid hydrolysis of the cellulose raw material for removing the bonded polysaccharides on cellulose fibril surface and a disordered or amorphous portion of cellulose that separates the fibrils (Revol et al. 1992). Acid hydrolysis is terminated by acid's rapid dilution, followed by the removal of acid via dialysis or centrifugation. Some mechanical forces like sonication are applied to terminate the aggregation of cellulose fibrils in order to yield cellulose nanocrystals having high crystallinity (Guo and Catchmark 2012). Cellulose nanocomposites show the different appearance from different sources, Figure 2 (Azizi Samir, Alloin, and Dufresne 2005).

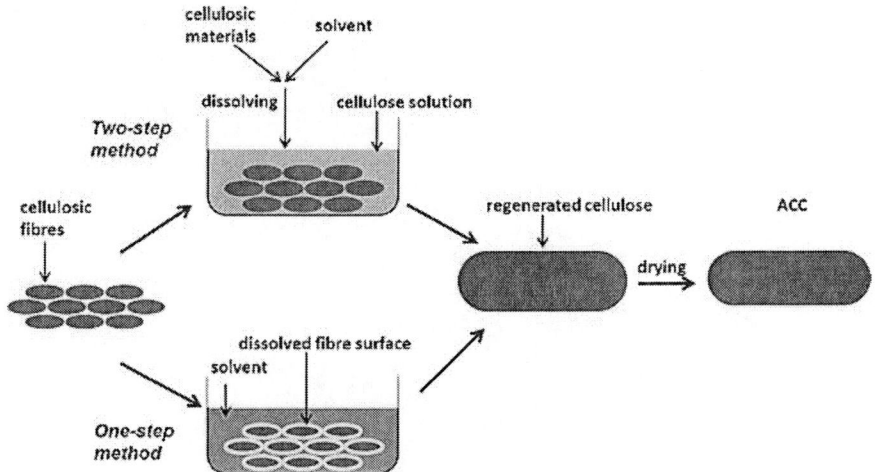

Figure 1. Schematic representation of the two-step (top) and one-step (bottom) preparation methods of ACCs Reprinted with permission from (Miao and Hamad 2013) Springer Nature, Cellulose, Cellulose reinforced polymer composites and nanocomposites: a critical review, Miao et al. 20 (2013) 2221-2262.

Favier (1995) first published the preparation of cellulose nanocrystals-reinforced polymer nanocomposites by using a latex which was achieved by the copolymerization of butyl acrylate (poly (S-co-BuA) and styrene and tunicin whiskers (the cellulose mined from tunicate-a sea animal). Numerous studies have been furnished on isolation and characterization of cellulose nanofibers due to in the development of nanocomposites, cellulose nanofibers have a great potential to be used in a various different area as reinforcement from various sources. These nanofibers can be extracted by only chemical or both chemical and mechanical methods from the cell walls (Alemdar and Sain 2008) Compatibility of fibers and polymers is a very common problem in cellulose fiber-based composites due to high polarity and hydrophilic nature of fibers but non-polar and hydrophobic nature of polymers. To overcome this problem surfaces of fibre can be treated using various methods such as physical (stretching (Haig Zeronian, Kawabata, and

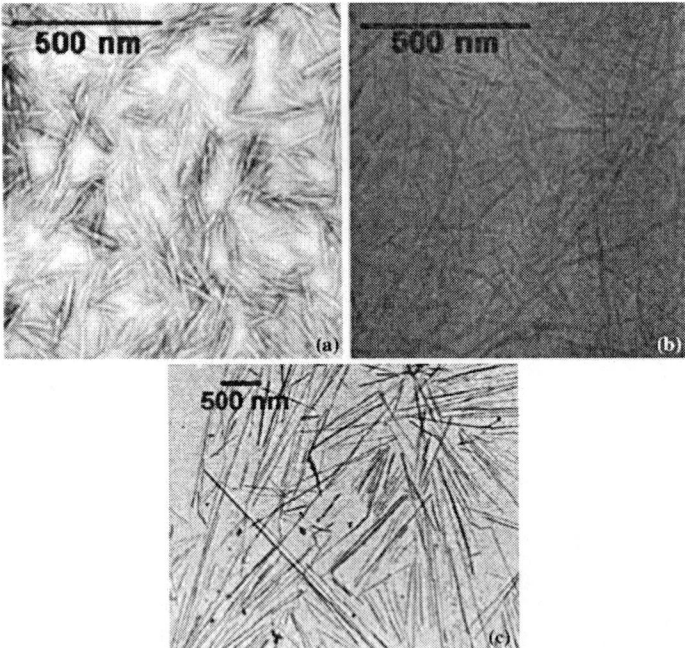

Figure 2. TEM images of CNC from different sources. a Cotton, b sugar-beet pulp, and c tunicin (the cellulose extracted from tunicate, a sea animal) Reprinted with permission from (Miao and Hamad 2013) Springer Nature, Cellulose, Cellulose reinforced polymer composites and nanocomposites: a critical review, Miao et al. 20 (2013) 2221-2262.

Alger 1990), calendering (Semsarzadeh 1986) and thermo-treatment Ray, Chakravarty, and Bandyopadhaya (1976), Physico-chemical (Takacs et al. 1999; Uehara and Sakata 1990; Carlsson and Stroem 1991; Kato et al. 1999; Kolar et al. 2000) and chemical methods (Belgacem and Gandini 2005). Various techniques can be used to characterize the modified fiber surface including scanning electron microscopy (SEM), X-ray photoelectron spectroscopy (XPS), Fourier transform infrared spectroscopy (FT-IR), contact angle measurements, confocal laser scanning microscopy (CLSM), elemental analysis, inverse gas chromatography (IGC), nuclear magnetic resonance (NMR) and atomic force microscopy (AFM) (Belgacem 2005; Mohanty, Misra, and Drzal 2001). Processing of cellulose nanofibers-reinforced nanocomposites by extrusion methods are explored rarely. The synthesis of cellulose nanocomposites by melt extrusion was prosecuted by injecting the suspension of nanocrystals into the polymer melt throughout the extrusion process (Oksman et al. 2006).

2.2. Properties of Cellulose Nanocomposites

2.2.1. Thermal Stability

Azizi Samir (2004) and Samir (2004) performed thermogravimetric analysis (TGA) experiments inspect the thermal degradation and stability of tunicin whiskers/POE nanocomposites and suggested that there was no effect of cellulosic fibers on POE nanocomposites degradation temperature. Choi and Simonsen (2006) suggested the effect of cotton cellulose nanocrystals content on the thermal behavior of CMC plasticized with glycerin revealed a close connotation between the filler and the matrix.

2.2.2. Mechanical Performance

Hajji (1996) studied the effect of preparation methods on the mechanical properties of a CNC-based nanocomposite. Nishino, Matsuda, and Hirao (2004) synthesized the cellulose nanocomposite films with cellulose I and II in the different ratio by the slight dissolution of microcrystalline cellulose powder in N, N-dimethylacetamide /lithium chloride and subsequent film casting and the structure and mechanical properties of these films were characterized by XRD and tensile strength. The resulting films are transparent to visible light, isotropic, highly crystalline having different amounts of undissolved cellulose I crystallites. By varying the cellulose I and II ratio, the mechanical recital of the nanocomposites can be tuned. studied The consequence of preparation or processing methods on the mechanical properties of a CNC-based nanocomposite was studied by Hajji (Hajji et al. 1996). He suggested that the composite film synthesized by water evaporation reveals the best mechanical property due to less impact on the orientation of CNC, offers better dispersion of CNC in matrices which safes CNC structure from damage. Hence, Table 1 shows the importance of processing methods and even dispersion of the reinforcement in the matrix on nanocomposite properties.

Table 1. Mechanical properties of CNC based nanocomposites processed by different methods (Miao and Hamad 2013) Reprinted with permission from Springer Nature, Cellulose, Cellulose reinforced polymer composites and nanocomposites: a critical review, Miao et al. 20 (2013) 2221-2262

CNC content (wt%)	E		HP		XP	
	Modulus (MPa)	Tensile strength (MPa)	Modulus (MPa)	Tensile strength (MPa)	Modulus (MPa)	Tensile strength (MPa)
0	0.2	0.15	0.2	0.12	0.2	0.12
1	0.6	0.49	0.5	0.31	0.4	0.23
6	32.3	5	5.2	1.63	1.5	1.06

The factors which affect the mechanical properties of cellulose nanocomposites are compatibility of polymer resin and CNC, the molecular structure of the matrix, the aspect ratio of CNC particles and composite preparation procedure.

3. APPLICATIONS

Application in the field of development of composites by cellulose nanofibers is a comparatively new research area. Eichhorn (2009) incorporated uses of cellulose-based nanocomposites in reinforce adhesives for making optically transparent paper designed for electronic display and to produce DNA-hybrid materials, to create hierarchical composites aimed to use in foams, aerogels and for improved coupling between fiber and matrix. Cellulose nanocomposites have proven to be an unusually multipurpose biomaterial that may be used in an extensive variety of applied scientific endeavors like electronics, paper products, acoustics, automotive industry and most important in pharmaceutical and biomedical devices.

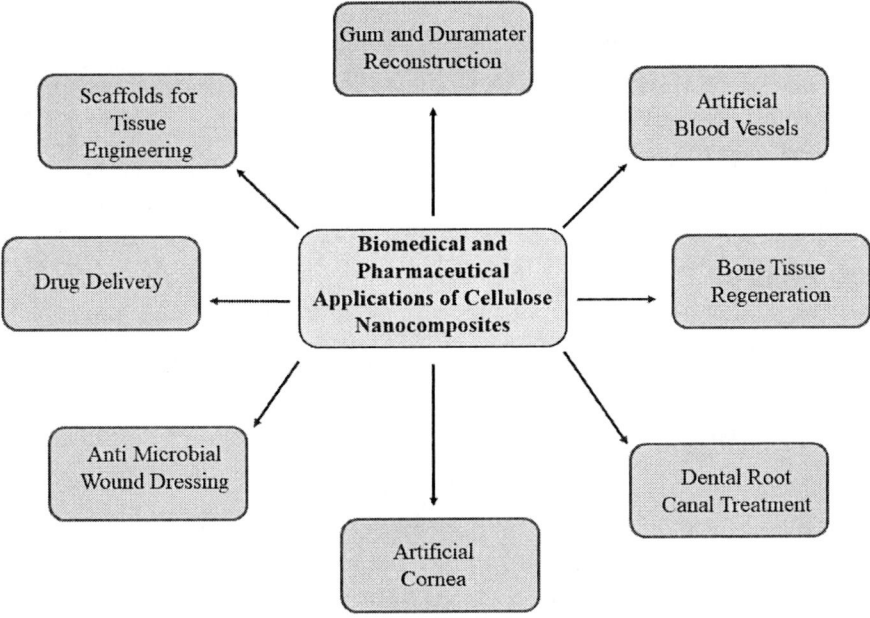

Figure 3. Biomedical and pharmaceutical applications of cellulose nanocomposites.

3.1. Pharmaceutical

Cellulose-based nanocomposites are highly useful in the pharmaceutical industry as cellulose has an outstanding property of compaction which blended smoothly with excipients in order to drug-loaded tablets form condensed matrices suitable for the oral management of drugs (Longer and Robinson 1990; Alderman 1984). Various potential advantages as a drug delivery excipient are offered by crystalline nanocellulose (Baumann et al. 2009; Watanabe et al. 2002). A large number of drugs can be found on the surface of cellulose nanocomposites due to high surface area along with the negative charge, makes them a potential candidate for high payloads and optimal control of dosing and it is also suitable because of established biocompatibility of cellulose. The hydroxyl groups present on the surface of crystalline nanocellulose offer a place for the surface amendment of the material with a wide range of chemical groups via many different methods. Modification of surface can be used to modulate the drug loading and release that would not normally tie to nanocellulose i.e., hydrophobic and nonionized. (Lönnberg et al. 2008; Shaikh et al. 2007).

3.2. Medical

Nowadays, eyes of biomaterial term has been used for nanocellulose because of its high applications in biomedical industry including drugs releasing system, skins replacements for wounds and burnings, nerves, blood vessel growth, scaffolds for tissue engineering, gum and dura mater reconstruction, stent covering and bone reconstruction (Mello et al. 2001; W. K. Czaja et al. 2007; Negrão et al. 2006; Klemm et al. 2001). Odontology is defied to find novel materials to substitute the bones in numerous procedures like facial deformities, maxillary, bone malformation and the loss of alveolar bone is the biggest challenge in this. Nanocellulose with appropriate porosity that provides the mat an infection barrier, painkiller effect, loss of fluids and allows medicines to be effortlessly applied and also works on purulent fluids by absorbing it during all inflammatory phases, ousting it later on in a painless and controlled manner (W. Czaja et al. 2006). Cellulose nanocomposites have all types of properties like physical, mechanical and chemical along with huge superficial areas that give outstanding water absorption capacity and also elasticity shows characteristics of an ideal healing bandage. Barud (2009) have developed a biological membrane with cellulose nanocomposites to standardized extract of propolis, it has several biological properties with anti-inflammatory and antimicrobial activities which makes the membrane for good treatment for chronic wounds and burns. Raghavendra (2013) reported the antibacterial activity of the cellulose nanocomposites against Escherichia coli which was done by inhibition zone method, suggested that the synthesized CSNCFs can function effectually as anti-microbial agents and can be used for tissue scaffolding.

3.3. Others

Other applications of nanocellulose composites are mainly focused on paper and packaging products as well as furniture, automotive, electronics, electroacoustic devices, construction, cosmetics, and pharmacy. Additionally, they are applied in ultrafiltration membranes (water purification), additives for a high-quality electronic paper (e-paper), membrane for combustible cells (hydrogen) and membranes used to retrieve mineral and oils (Brown 1998). The high stiffness and strength along with the small dimensions of nanocellulose may enhanced properties to composite materials reinforced with cellulose fibers and these could afterward be used in wide range of applications. Cellulose nanocomposites have been used in audio diaphragms due to its property to bear two essential properties that are low dynamic loss and high sonic velocity. It is stated that the sonic velocity of films was virtually equivalent to those of titanium and aluminum (Iguchi, Yamanaka, and Budhiono 2000). Jonas and Farah (1998) reported that SONY had already been using it in headphones diaphragm. In Kyoto University, researchers prepared strong but enhanced transparent composite material by isolating nanofibrillated cellulose structure by improving the dispersion of nanofibers in the matrix and on this basis, an organic display system is being developed recently (Shimazaki et al. 2007; Iwamoto et al. 2005).

CONCLUSION

Cellulose nanocomposites are unique nanomaterials derived from most abundant natural polymer, cellulose, which is made from superfine fibrils in nanoscale diameters. It has been observed that from last 15 years there has been steady progress in the field of cellulosic nanocomposites. Cellulose nanofibers have exciting potential to be used as reinforcement in nanocomposites as these are non-toxic, sustainable, renewable and biocompatible nanomaterials. The present chapter gives an overview of the use of cellulose fibers as reinforcement material in polymer matrices. The aim of chapter is to provide knowledge of cellulose nanocomposites for further research and studies. The chapter also summarizes the effect of processing methods and other parameters on thermal and mechanical properties of nanocomposites. The potential mechanical properties of cellulose nanocomposites vie well with other engineering materials and devices. Processing methods, properties, and applications in various fields such as pharmaceutical, medical and others are well discussed in the chapter.

REFERENCES

Alderman, D A. 1984. "A Review of Cellulose Ethers in Hydrophilic Matrices for Oral Controlled-Release Dosage Forms." *Int J Pharm Tech Prod Mfr* 5 (3): 1–9.

Alemdar, Ayse, and Mohini Sain. 2008. "Biocomposites from Wheat Straw Nanofibers: Morphology, Thermal and Mechanical Properties." *Composites Science and Technology* 68 (2). Elsevier: 557–65.

Azizi Samir, My Ahmed Said, Fannie Alloin, and Alain Dufresne. 2005. "Review of Recent Research into Cellulosic Whiskers, Their Properties and Their Application in Nanocomposite Field." *Biomacromolecules* 6 (2). ACS Publications: 612–26.

Azizi Samir, My Ahmed Said, Fannie Alloin, Wladimir Gorecki, Jean-Yves Sanchez, and Alain Dufresne. 2004. "Nanocomposite Polymer Electrolytes Based on Poly (Oxyethylene) and Cellulose Nanocrystals." *The Journal of Physical Chemistry B* 108 (30). ACS Publications: 10845–52.

Barud, H S. 2009. "Development and Evaluation of Biocure Obtained from Bacterial Cellulose and Standardized Extract of Propolis (EPP-AF) for the Treatment of Burns and/or Skin Lesions." *Sao Paulo Research Foundation—FAPESP, Brazil*.

Baumann, M Douglas, Catherine E Kang, Jason C Stanwick, Yuanfei Wang, Howard Kim, Yakov Lapitsky, and Molly S Shoichet. 2009. "An Injectable Drug Delivery Platform for Sustained Combination Therapy." *Journal of Controlled Release* 138 (3). Elsevier: 205–13.

Belgacem, Mohamed Naceur. 2005. "The Surface Modification of Cellulose Fibres in View of Their Use as Reinforcing Elements in Composite Materials." In *Last Developments in Pulp Bleaching, Ozone Bleaching, Chemical Modification of Fibers EFPG Days*.

Belgacem, Mohamed Naceur, and Alessandro Gandini. 2005. "The Surface Modification of Cellulose Fibres for Use as Reinforcing Elements in Composite Materials." *Composite Interfaces* 12 (1–2). Taylor & Francis: 41–75.

Berglund, Lars A, and Ton Peijs. 2010. "Cellulose Biocomposites—from Bulk Moldings to Nanostructured Systems." *MRS Bulletin* 35 (3). Cambridge University Press: 201–7.

Bledzki, A K, S Reihmane, and J Gassan. 1996. "Properties and Modification Methods for Vegetable Fibers for Natural Fiber Composites." *Journal of Applied Polymer Science* 59 (8). Wiley Online Library: 1329–36.

Bondeson, Daniel, and Kristiina Oksman. 2007. "Dispersion and Characteristics of Surfactant Modified Cellulose Whiskers Nanocomposites." *Composite Interfaces* 14 (7–9). Taylor & Francis: 617–30.

Booker, Richard D, and Earl Boysen. 2005. *Nanotechnology for Dummies*. John Wiley & Sons.

Brown, R M. 1998. "Microbial Cellulose: A New Resource for Wood, Paper, Textiles, Food and Specialty Products." *Position Paper*.

Carlsson, C M Gilbert, and Goeran Stroem. 1991. "Reduction and Oxidation of Cellulose Surfaces by Means of Cold Plasma." *Langmuir* 7 (11). ACS Publications: 2492–97.

Chazeau, Laurent, J Y Cavaille, G Canova, R Dendievel, and B Boutherin. 1999. "Viscoelastic Properties of Plasticized PVC Reinforced with Cellulose Whiskers." *Journal of Applied Polymer Science* 71 (11). Wiley Online Library: 1797–1808.

Chen, Jinhua, and Norio Tsubokawa. 2000. "Electric Properties of Conducting Composite from Poly (Ethylene Oxide) and Poly (Ethylene Oxide)-Grafted Carbon Black in Solvent Vapor." *Polymer Journal* 32 (9). Nature Publishing Group: 729.

Choi, YongJae, and John Simonsen. 2006. "Cellulose Nanocrystal-Filled Carboxymethyl Cellulose Nanocomposites." *Journal of Nanoscience and Nanotechnology* 6 (3). American Scientific Publishers: 633–39.

Crawford, Ronald L. 1981. *Lignin Biodegradation and Transformation*. John Wiley and Sons.

Czaja, Wojciech K, David J Young, Marek Kawecki, and R Malcolm Brown. 2007. "The Future Prospects of Microbial Cellulose in Biomedical Applications." *Biomacromolecules* 8 (1). ACS Publications: 1–12.

Czaja, Wojciech, Alina Krystynowicz, Stanislaw Bielecki, and R Malcolm Brown Jr. 2006. "Microbial Cellulose—the Natural Power to Heal Wounds." *Biomaterials* 27 (2). Elsevier: 145–51.

Dorée, Charles. 1947. "The Methods of Cellulose Chemistry Including Methods for the Investigation of Substances Associated with Cellulose in Plant Tissues." *The Methods of Cellulose Chemistry Including Methods for the Investigation of Substances Associated with Cellulose in Plant Tissues.*, no. Edn 2 (revised). Chapman and Hall, Ltd.

Eichhorn, S J, A Dufresne, M Aranguren, N E Marcovich, J R Capadona, S J Rowan, C Weder, et al. 2009. "Review: Current International Research into Cellulose Nanofibres and Nanocomposites." *Journal of Materials Science* 45 (1): 1. doi:10.1007/s10853-009-3874-0.

Favier, V, G R Canova, J Y Cavaillé, H Chanzy, A Dufresne, and C Gauthier. 1995. "Nanocomposite Materials from Latex and Cellulose Whiskers." *Polymers for Advanced Technologies* 6 (5). Wiley Online Library: 351–55.

Fu, Lian-Hua, Chao Qi, Ming-Guo Ma, and Pengbo Wan. 2019. "Multifunctional Cellulose-Based Hydrogels for Biomedical Applications." *Journal of Materials Chemistry B*. The Royal Society of Chemistry. doi:10.1039/C8TB02331J.

Gindl, W, and J Keckes. 2005. "All-Cellulose Nanocomposite." *Polymer* 46 (23). Elsevier: 10221–25.

Guo, Jing, and Jeffrey M Catchmark. 2012. "Surface Area and Porosity of Acid Hydrolyzed Cellulose Nanowhiskers and Cellulose Produced by Gluconacetobacter Xylinus." *Carbohydrate Polymers* 87 (2). Elsevier: 1026–37.

Haig Zeronian, S, Hiroko Kawabata, and Kenneth W Alger. 1990. "Factors Affecting the Tensile Properties of Nonmercerized and Mercerized Cotton Fibers." *Textile Research Journal* 60 (3). Sage Publications Sage CA: Thousand Oaks, CA: 179–83.

Hajji, P, J Y Cavaille, V Favier, C Gauthier, and G Vigier. 1996. "Tensile Behavior of Nanocomposites from Latex and Cellulose Whiskers." *Polymer Composites* 17 (4). Wiley Online Library: 612–19.

Hamad, Wadood Y. 2013. *Cellulosic Materials: Fibers, Networks and Composites*. Springer Science & Business Media.

Henriksson, Marielle, Gunnar Henriksson, L A Berglund, and Tom Lindström. 2007. "An Environmentally Friendly Method for Enzyme-Assisted Preparation of Microfibrillated Cellulose (MFC) Nanofibers." *European Polymer Journal* 43 (8). Elsevier: 3434–41.

Hornsby, P R, E Hinrichsen, and K Tarverdi. 1997. "Preparation and Properties of Polypropylene Composites Reinforced with Wheat and Flax Straw Fibres: Part II Analysis of Composite Microstructure and Mechanical Properties." *Journal of Materials Science* 32 (4). Springer: 1009–15.

Iguchi, M, S Yamanaka, and A Budhiono. 2000. "Bacterial Cellulose—a Masterpiece of Nature's Arts." *Journal of Materials Science* 35 (2). Springer: 261–70.

Iwamoto, Shinichiro, Antonio Norio Nakagaito, Hiroyuki Yano, and Masaya Nogi. 2005. "Optically Transparent Composites Reinforced with Plant Fiber-Based Nanofibers." *Applied Physics A* 81 (6). Springer: 1109–12.

Jonas, Rainer, and Luiz F Farah. 1998. "Production and Application of Microbial Cellulose." *Polymer Degradation and Stability* 59 (1–3). Elsevier: 101–6.

Kalia, Susheel, Alain Dufresne, Bibin Mathew Cherian, B S Kaith, Luc Avérous, James Njuguna, and Elias Nassiopoulos. 2011. "Cellulose-Based Bio-and Nanocomposites: A Review." *International Journal of Polymer Science* 2011. Hindawi.

Kato, Koichi, Victor N Vasilets, Mikhail N Fursa, Masashi Meguro, Yoshito Ikada, and Katsuhiko Nakamae. 1999. "Surface Oxidation of Cellulose Fibers by Vacuum Ultraviolet Irradiation." *Journal of Polymer Science Part A: Polymer Chemistry* 37 (3). Wiley Online Library: 357–61.

Klemm, Dieter, Dieter Schumann, Ulrike Udhardt, and Silvia Marsch. 2001. "Bacterial Synthesized Cellulose—artificial Blood Vessels for Microsurgery." *Progress in Polymer Science* 26 (9). Elsevier: 1561–1603.

Kolar, Jana, Matija Strlic, Doris Müller-Hess, Andreas Gruber, Karin Troschke, Simone Pentzien, and Wolfgang Kautek. 2000. "Near-UV and Visible Pulsed Laser Interaction with Paper." *Journal of Cultural Heritage* 1. Elsevier: S221–24.

Kvien, Ingvild, Junji Sugiyama, Martin Votrubec, and Kristiina Oksman. 2007. "Characterization of Starch Based Nanocomposites." *Journal of Materials Science* 42 (19). Springer: 8163–71.

Longer, Mark A, and Joseph R Robinson. 1990. "Sustained-Release Drug Delivery Systems." *Remington's Pharmaceutical Sciences* 18. Mack Publishing Easton, PA: 20.

Lönnberg, Hanna, Linda Fogelström, My Ahmed Said Azizi Samir, Lars Berglund, Eva Malmström, and Anders Hult. 2008. "Surface Grafting of Microfibrillated Cellulose with Poly (ε-Caprolactone)–Synthesis and Characterization." *European Polymer Journal* 44 (9). Elsevier: 2991–97.

Lu, Wei, Hongfei Lin, and Guohua Chen. 2007. "Voltage-induced Resistivity Relaxation in a High-density Polyethylene/Graphite Nanosheet Composite." *Journal of Polymer Science Part B: Polymer Physics* 45 (7). Wiley Online Library: 860–63.

Mello, Luis Renato, Yanara Feltrin, Rafael Selbach, Gilberto Macedo Junior, Cleverton Spautz, and Leandro José Haas. 2001. "Use of Lyophilized Cellulose in Peripheral Nerve Lesions with Loss of Substance." *Arquivos de Neuro-Psiquiatria* 59 (2B). SciELO Brasil: 372–79.

Miao, Chuanwei, and Wadood Y Hamad. 2013. "Cellulose Reinforced Polymer Composites and Nanocomposites: A Critical Review." *Cellulose* 20 (5): 2221–62. doi:10.1007/s10570-013-0007-3.

Mohanty, A K, Manjusri Misra, and Lawrence T Drzal. 2001. "Surface Modifications of Natural Fibers and Performance of the Resulting Biocomposites: An Overview." *Composite Interfaces* 8 (5). Taylor & Francis: 313–43.

Negrão, Stefan Wolanski, Ronaldo da Rocha Loures Bueno, E E Guérios, Frederico Thomaz Ultramari, Alysson Moço Faidiga, Paulo Maurício Piá de Andrade, Déborah Christina Nercolini, José Carlos Tarastchuck, and Luiz Fernando Farah. 2006. "A Eficácia Do Stent Recoberto Com Celulose Biossintética Comparado Ao Stent Convencional Em Angioplastia Em Coelhos." *Revista Brasileira de Cardiologia Invasiva* 14 (1): 10–19.

Nishino, Takashi, Ikuyo Matsuda, and Koichi Hirao. 2004. "All-Cellulose Composite." *Macromolecules* 37 (20). ACS Publications: 7683–87.

Oksman, Kristiina, Aji P Mathew, Daniel Bondeson, and Ingvild Kvien. 2006. "Manufacturing Process of Cellulose Whiskers/Polylactic Acid Nanocomposites." *Composites Science and Technology* 66 (15). Elsevier: 2776–84.

Oksman, Kristiina, Lennart Wallström, Lars A Berglund, and Romildo Dias Toledo Filho. 2002. "Morphology and Mechanical Properties of

Unidirectional Sisal–epoxy Composites." *Journal of Applied Polymer Science* 84 (13). Wiley Online Library: 2358–65.

Payen, Anselme. 1838. "Mémoire Sur La Composition Du Tissu Propre Des Plantes et Du Ligneux." *Comptes Rendus* 7: 1052–56.

Raghavendra, Gownolla Malegowd, Tippabattini Jayaramudu, Kokkarachedu Varaprasad, Rotimi Sadiku, S Sinha Ray, and Konduru Mohana Raju. 2013. "Cellulose–polymer–Ag Nanocomposite Fibers for Antibacterial Fabrics/Skin Scaffolds." *Carbohydrate Polymers* 93 (2): 553–60. doi:https://doi.org/10.1016/j.carbpol.2012.12.035.

Ranby, Bengt G. 1952. "The Cellulose Micelles." *Tappi* 35 (2). TAPPI PRESS TECH ASSN PULP & PAPER IND 1 DUNWOODY PARK, ATLANTA, GA 30338: 53–58.

Rånby, Bengt G. 1951. "Fibrous Macromolecular Systems. Cellulose and Muscle. The Colloidal Properties of Cellulose Micelles." *Discussions of the Faraday Society* 11. Royal Society of Chemistry: 158–64.

Ray, P K, A C Chakravarty, and S B Bandyopadhaya. 1976. "Fine Structure and Mechanical Properties of Jute Differently Dried after Retting." *Journal of Applied Polymer Science* 20 (7). Wiley Online Library: 1765–67.

Revol, J-F, H Bradford, J Giasson, R H Marchessault, and D G Gray. 1992. "Helicoidal Self-Ordering of Cellulose Microfibrils in Aqueous Suspension." *International Journal of Biological Macromolecules* 14 (3). Elsevier: 170–72.

Samir, My Ahmed Said Azizi, Fannie Alloin, Jean-Yves Sanchez, and Alain Dufresne. 2004. "Cellulose Nanocrystals Reinforced Poly (Oxyethylene)." *Polymer* 45 (12). Elsevier: 4149–57.

Semsarzadeh, Mohammad A. 1986. "Fiber Matrix Interactions in Jute Reinforced Polyester Resin." *Polymer Composites* 7 (1). Wiley Online Library: 23–25.

Setua, D K, and S K De. 1984. "Short Silk Fibre Reinforced Nitrile Rubber Composites." *Journal of Materials Science* 19 (3). Springer: 983–99.

Shaikh, Sohel, Anil Birdi, Syed Qutubuddin, Eric Lakatosh, and Harihara Baskaran. 2007. "Controlled Release in Transdermal Pressure Sensitive

Adhesives Using Organosilicate Nanocomposites." *Annals of Biomedical Engineering* 35 (12). Springer: 2130–37.

Shimazaki, Yuzuru, Yasuo Miyazaki, Yoshitaka Takezawa, Masaya Nogi, Kentaro Abe, Shinsuke Ifuku, and Hiroyuki Yano. 2007. "Excellent Thermal Conductivity of Transparent Cellulose Nanofiber/Epoxy Resin Nanocomposites." *Biomacromolecules* 8 (9). ACS Publications: 2976–78.

Sorrentino, Andrea, Giuliana Gorrasi, and Vittoria Vittoria. 2007. "Potential Perspectives of Bio-Nanocomposites for Food Packaging Applications." *Trends in Food Science & Technology* 18 (2). Elsevier: 84–95.

Takacs, E, L Wojnárovits, J Borsa, Cs Földváry, P Hargittai, and O Zöld. 1999. "Effect of γ-Irradiation on Cotton-Cellulose." *Radiation Physics and Chemistry* 55 (5–6). Elsevier: 663–66.

Uehara, Tohru, and Isao Sakata. 1990. "Effect of Corona Discharge Treatment on Cellulose Prepared from Beech Wood." *Journal of Applied Polymer Science* 41 (7-8). Wiley Online Library: 1695–1706.

Vallejos, María E, Maria S Peresin, and Orlando J Rojas. 2012. "All-Cellulose Composite Fibers Obtained by Electrospinning Dispersions of Cellulose Acetate and Cellulose Nanocrystals." *Journal of Polymers and the Environment* 20 (4). Springer: 1075–83.

Vilay, V, M Mariatti, R Mat Taib, and Mitsugu Todo. 2008. "Effect of Fiber Surface Treatment and Fiber Loading on the Properties of Bagasse Fiber–reinforced Unsaturated Polyester Composites." *Composites Science and Technology* 68 (3–4). Elsevier: 631–38.

Watanabe, Yoshiteru, Baku Mukai, Ken-ichi Kawamura, Tatsuya Ishikawa, Michihiro Namiki, Naoki Utoguchi, and Makiko Fujii. 2002. "Preparation and Evaluation of Press-Coated Aminophylline Tablet Using Crystalline Cellulose and Polyethylene Glycol in the Outer Shell for Timed-Release Dosage Forms." *Yakugaku Zasshi: Journal of the Pharmaceutical Society of Japan* 122 (2): 157–62.

Zárate, C N, M I Aranguren, and M M Reboredo. 2008. "Thermal Degradation of a Phenolic Resin, Vegetable Fibers, and Derived Composites." *Journal of Applied Polymer Science* 107 (5). Wiley Online Library: 2977–85.

Zhou, Yuanxin, Farhana Pervin, Vijaya K Rangari, and Shaik Jeelani. 2006. "Fabrication and Evaluation of Carbon Nano Fiber Filled Carbon/Epoxy Composite." *Materials Science and Engineering: A* 426 (1–2). Elsevier: 221–28.

In: Biocomposites in Bio-Medicine
Editors: Mudasir Ahmad et al.
ISBN: 978-1-53616-247-9
© 2019 Nova Science Publishers, Inc.

Chapter 3

APPLICATION OF GELATIN IN BIOMEDICAL FIELD

Shikha Gupta[*]
School of Basic & Applied Sciences, Department of Chemistry,
Lingaya's Vidyapeeth, Faridabad, Haryana, India

ABSTRACT

Gelatin is remarkably known for its various merits like biodegradability, biocompatibility, availability at low cost and ease of processing, because of these properties it has been widely used in pharmaceutical formulation, tissue engineering and in cell culture. In addition, gelatin can also be used for ocular applications, bio-adhesives, and bio-artificial grafts. These different applications have diverse physical, chemical and biological requirements and this has prompted research into the modification of gelatin and its derivatives. It differs from other hydrocolloids because most of them are polysaccharides, whereas gelatin is a digestible protein containing all the essential amino acids. In this chapter, we discuss the uses of gelatin in various biomedical fields.

Keywords: gelatin, biomedical, tissue engineering, artificial grafts

---

[*] Corresponding Author's Email: shika641@gmail.com.

1. Introduction

Gelatin is a natural, biodegradable, biocompatible and multifunctional biopolymer. It is extracted mainly from cattle bones, hide, pork skin and fishes. Depending upon the method of collagen hydrolysis they are of two types "type A and type B". Type A gelatin is obtained by acid hydrolysis of gelatin. Acid processing barely affects the amide groups of glutamine and asparagine, resulting in a higher isoelectric point (IEP), i.e., 7-9 (Patel et al. 2008). Type B gelatin derived by alkaline hydrolyzes of asparagine and glutamine to aspartate and glutamate, respectively. Thus it possesses a greater proportion of carboxyl groups, rendering it negatively charged and lowering its IEP (i.e., 4.5 - 6.0) (Ninan et al. 2011). As a protein, gelatin exhibits an amphoteric behavior due to the presence of both acidic and basic functional groups, as a result of existence of amino acid functional groups and terminal amino and carboxyl groups. It differs from other hydrocolloids because most of them are polysaccharide, whereas gelatin is a digestible protein containing all the essential amino acids except tryptophan (Mariod et al. 2013). It contains approximately 20 amino acids which are linked together in a partially ordered fashion. Four groups of amino acids are predominant in the gelatin molecule. In every 1000 residues of gelatin's amino acid residues, 330 are glycine, 132 are proline, 112 are alanine, 93 are hydroxyproline and the rest are other residues (Schrieber et al. 2007). The triple helical structure of gelatin is due to Glycine X-Proline, where X represents the amino acids like lysine, arginine, methionine, and valine. Glycine, being dominant component, is the smallest amino acid as its lateral group is hydrogen. Pro and Hypro—with rigid lateral pyrrolidine rings—display steric hindrances (Hoque et al. 2015). A typical structure of gelatin shows Ala-Gly-Pro-Arg-Gly-Glu-4Hyp-Gly-Pro- arrangement (Figure 1). Moreover, chemical composition and distribution of particular amino acids may affect rigidity of gelatin chain. Each amino acid chain may have a molecular weight between 10,000 and several hundred thousands of Daltons, depending upon the raw material and conditions of the conversion of collagen into gelatin. The surface property of gelatin is a polyampholyte.

However, the gelatin is negatively charged at higher pH and positively charged at lower pH.

Gelatin is remarkably known for its various merits which makes it a versatile natural biopolymer like it is cheap, widely available, denatured product and it is much less antigenic than collagen. The gelatin chains contain abundant amino sequences that modulate cell adhesion, thereby improving the final biological behavior over polymers that lack these cell-recognition sites (Wang et al. 2012). The diverse and accessible functional groups of gelatin allow for chemical modifications, such as coupling with cross-linkers and targeting-ligands. It also provides intermediate structural support when blending with other material constituents (Tang et al. 2012). At temperature > 35 - 40°C gelatin-water mixture exists as a sol (Tanaka et al. 2003). At further lower temperature the intramolecular hydrogen bonding induces a transition from sol to a structured three-dimensional gel, at concentration higher than approximately 1% (Gao et al. 2014). Lower concentration does not have sufficient molecules to support an infinite three-dimensional gel network (Parker and Povey 2012).

Being a versatile natural polymer, gelatin is widely used in food, photographic, medical, cosmetic and pharmaceutical products. In the food products, it is utilized as a film former, the gelling agent providing texture and shape to food (Cheng et al. 2014; Hanani et al. 2014). In the medical field and pharmaceutical fields, gelatin is currently used as in tissue engineering (Su and Wang 2015) as a matrix for implants, device coatings and as a stabilizer in vaccines against measles, mumps, rubella, Japanese encephalitis, rabies, diphtheria and tetanus toxin (Burke et al. 1999; Fooxand Meital2015). It is also used in intravenous infusions, hard and soft capsules, plasma expanders, wound dressings, tissue bio-adhesives, hemostats, sealants and in drug delivery systems (Karimand Bhat 2009; Panduranga 1996; Pollack 1990; Saddler and Horsey 1987). Due to its innate properties it has gained new interests in drug delivery systems (Santoro et al. 2014) such as hydrogels (Cui et al. 2014), films (Li et al. 20140, microcapsules (Prataand Grosso 2015), nanoparticles, etc. (Abrams et al. 2006; Rajan and Raj 2013; Azimi et al. 2014; Khan 2014).

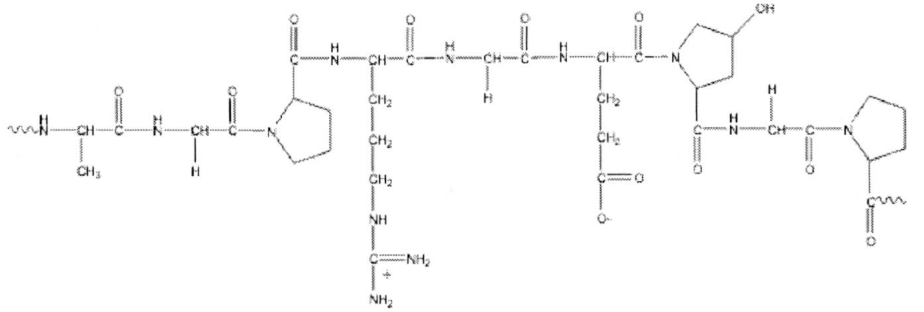

Figure 1. Structure of gelatin representing; Ala-Gly-Pro-Arg-Gly-Glu-4Hyp-Gly-Pro units.

2. APPLICATION OF GELATIN

Gelatin dissolves rapidly in the water at 37°C, non-immunogenic, and fully absorbable polymer. These properties have attracted the researchers to use gelatin in biomedical field. In this chapter we focused on the various applications of gelatin in the biomedical field.

2.1. Cardiovascular

Gelatin is an attractive biopolymer and has been used as a suitable scaffolding biomaterial for cardiovascular tissue engineering. Recent advances in the tissue engineering field have attracted significant attention in creating cardiac tissue concepts. Hydrogels, porous and fibrous frameworks are used in cardiac tissue engineering (Raneand Christman2011). For example, commercially available gelatin-based foams (e.g., Gelfoam®, water-insoluble gelatin sponge) have been planted with cells derived from fetal rat ventricular muscle to form functional cardiac grafts (Li et al. 1999). The results of this study show that the cells are able to grow and instinctively exhausted within the 3D microenvironment of the gelatin matrix, in both *in vitro* and *in vivo* (implantation) studies. Gelatin has been also mixed with other synthetic biomaterials such as polycaprolactone (PCL), polylactic acid (PLA), and poly (glycerol-sebacate) (PGS) for creating frameworks with adjustable degradation rate and desired mechanical properties to control cellular organization and impersonator the grading of the native cardiac tissue (Li et al. 2000; Ozawa et al. 2004; Ifkovits et al. 2009; Kharaziha et al. 2013; Nerurkar et al. 2007; Tamayol et al. 2013). Since gelatin is an insulating biopolymer, conductive nanoparticles such as carbon nanotubes (CNTs) have been incorporated into photo cross-linkable GelMA hydrogel to enhance the electrical and mechanical properties of the tissue matrix and improve spontaneous beating of cardiomyocytes as compared to pure gelatin hydrogel.

By using photolithography a highly organized endothelial cord-like structures within GelMA hydrogel can be created (Nikkhah et al. 2012). It is also proven that the dimensions of the micropatterned features significantly affected proliferation, alignment, and cord formation of the encapsulated endothelial cells. In another study, co-culture of mesenchymal stem cells (MSCs) and endothelial progenitor cells (EPCs) inside Gel-MA (Methacrylated gelatin) hydrogel of different methacrylation degrees resulted in the extensive formation of biomimetic capillary networks (Chen et al. 2012). An electrospun scaffold made with the blend of gelatin, poly (lactic-co-glycolic acid) (PLGA) and elastin has also shown a great promise as suitable biomaterials for vascular tissue engineering (Han et al. 2010).

2.2. Drug Delivery

Gelatin has been extensively investigated as a drug delivery carrier due to its properties and history of safe use in a wide range of medical applications. Gelatin's properties can be modified and adjusted to maximize drug loading and efficiency of release for many classes of drugs. Incorporating bioactive molecules into appropriate carriers offers many advantages compared to conventional dosage forms. It can improve patient compliance and convenience by reducing possible toxic side effects of the drug. The release profile from gelatin carriers were shown to be optimized by changing the gelatin source, its molecular weight and the degree of its crosslinking. The amount of loaded drug and the type of interaction between the drug and the carrier depending on the chemical structure of the drug and the carrier and the conditions of the drug-loading procedure. Gelatin microparticles and nanoparticles have been widely used for encapsulating many bioactive molecules. Microparticles have a relatively large surface area and can, therefore, serve as vehicles for cell strengthening and in distribution of large bioactive molecules to the desired site. Nanoparticles have a higher intracellular uptake and are better suited for intravenous or drug delivery in different areas in the body. Due to their unique design, liposomes have the ability to incorporate both hydrophilic and hydrophobic drugs, protect them from degradation, target them to the desired site and reduce the toxicity or side effects of those molecules. Embedding liposomes into a gelatin-based system resulted in an improvement in their stability and viscosity and in the half-life of the loaded drug and the liposome. As a drug carrier, gelatin fibers contain a high surface area to volume ratio, high porosity, and controllable pore size and can, therefore, accelerate the solubility of the drug in the aqueous solution and enhance the drug's efficiency. Gelatin hydrogels can trap molecules within the gaps between the polymer crosslinks. In the body, due to direct contact with water, they swell and the gaps between the polymer crosslinks increase, allowing the drugs to diffuse into the bloodstream. However, work is continually being carried out in order to improve gelatin release technology by modification of gelatin to allow the release of a wider variety of biomolecules from gelatin carriers for a broad range of applications (Foox and Zilberman 2015).

2.3. Bone Tissue Engineering

Bone is a hard, solid connective tissue that provides structure and protection to the body. To support external loading and absorb shocks, bone has a unique structure and chemical composition. Bone formation is a highly complex and dynamic process, (Hoque et al. 2015) which initially starts with recruitment of osteoprogenitor cells. The bone structure is composed of two layers of different density of bones. The outer layer is compact bone and the inner layer being spongy bone. Bone is always undergoing dynamic remodeling carried out by two different cell types, the osteoblast for building bone and the osteoclast for digesting bone (Bose et al. 2012). Bone defects are common diseases and the number of patients suffering from this condition keeps increasing. Scaffolds utilizing natural and synthetic polymers combined with bone cells are seen as a promising approach to overcome the limitation of the conventional treatment for bone defects. A study shows that (Pereira et al. 2014) the osteogenic differentiation and proliferation of human adipose-derived stem cells (hASCs) on the mineralized PCL-GE (Polycaprolactone- Gelatin) scaffolds are considered to be of great importance in bone tissue engineering. In another study, (Wen et al. 2013) found that the umbilical cord-derived mesenchymal stem cells (hUC-MSCs) exhibited bone regeneration potential with strong expression of specific osteogenic markers *in vitro*. Moreover, the hUC-MSCs also displayed faster proliferation which provides a larger number of cells in short time period to meet the needs of bone tissue engineering. In other words gelatin-based scaffolds and microspheres were meant for sequential release of growth factors to initiate bone regeneration and improve vascularization at the injury site (Kempen et al. 2009; Patel et al. 2008). Alternatively, others have proposed the use of gelatin hydrogels for ex vivo gene transfer aiding bone regeneration (Kim et al. 2004). Beyond these applications, gelatin-based scaffolds have been used to decrease bacterial bone infections through the sustained release of antibiotics and antimicrobial agents post-fracture or implantation (Kuijpers et al. 1998; Di Silvio and Bonfield, 1999; Yaffe et al. 2003).

2.4. Cosmetics

Skin is the largest tissue covering the body and provides physical and chemical protection of the body from harmful sources such as heat and microbial organisms (Li 2007). The skin has two layers; the epidermis or outer layer, which is constantly regenerated, and the dermis on the inner layer that provides mechanical support for the dermis (Hench and Jones 2005). Gelatin, which is a denatured derivative of collagen, has been shown to be a promising biomaterial for creating skin grafts (Metcalfe and Ferguson 2006). For instance, gelatin has been extensively used alone (Lee et al. 2005; Perng et al. 2008; Powell and Boyce 2008) or in combination with other natural and synthetic biomaterials. Few studies showed, a good affinity of the human dermal fibroblast (HDF) on the pure gelatin scaffolds even after treated with GTA (Glutaraldehyde) (Zhang et al. 2006). However, initial inhibition of cell proliferation was observed, possibly due to the existence of residual GTA. The blend of gelatin with other natural polymer has been demonstrated in many studies to promote the cell growth and proliferation of the HDF. It is found that the blends of gelatin with natural polymers exhibit better support for cell attachment, adhesion, and proliferation (Vatankhah et al. 2014). On the other side, the higher concentration of gelatin in the blend is unfavorable for growth of fibroblasts. It was found that high concentration of gelatin reduced the scaffold porosity which eventually unfavorable for cell growth (Enrione et al. 2013). To improve on the cell growth, have impregnated collagen-gelatin scaffold with basic fibroblast growth factor (bFGF) to accelerate skin regeneration (Ayvazyan et al. 2011). However, blends of gelatin-natural polymer display poor mechanical properties, especially under wet conditions. Whereas, the blend of gelatin and synthetic polymers were found to enhance the biomechanical properties of the scaffold. When human keratinocytes seeded on gelatin-PCL (polycaprolactone) scaffolds showed good biocompatibility and found to accelerate the wound closure progress (Morimoto et al. 2013). Collagen type I when incorporated on the surface of gelatin-PCL scaffold, the cell adherence, proliferation, and migration of the fibroblast was greater (Duan et al. 2013). Another polymer that is frequently blended with gelatin is a PHB (Poly (3-hydroxybutyric acid) a hydrophobic polymer-supported the adhesion and proliferation of HDFs and keratinocytes with a prolonged half-life *in vivo* (Gautam et al. 2014; Nagiah et al. 2013).

2.5. Wound Dressings

Wound care materials should provide a warm and moist environment for a rapid healing process; in addition, they should prevent the proliferation of bacteria around the wound area (Winter 1962; Barnett and Irving 1991; Choi et al. 1999). Consequently, wound dressing hydrogels with biodegradability, good fluid absorbance, transparency, and optimal water vapor permeability are preferred over the preformed dressings (e.g., commercial dressings in the forms of membranes and sheets) for the wound healing process (Jaipan et al. 2017). Oxidized alginate- and gelatin-based hydrogel when used for wound dressing application via *in vivo* study in a rat model shows promising results with relatively low water vapor transmission rate compared with commercially available wound dressing products and good water absorptivity. The improved water retention facilitated the development of a moist environment that is conducive to wound healing; the alginate- and gelatin-based hydrogel was shown to enhance cell migration and re-epithelialization (Balakrishnan et al. 2005). Dextran dialdehyde cross-linked gelatin hydrogel is also used for wound dressing material (Draye et al. 1998). Gelatin-based hydrogel sheets with high antibacterial efficacy have also been fabricated from gelatin, honey, and chitosan (Wang et al. 2012). *In vitro* and *in vivo* studies demonstrated that these sheets did not exhibit toxic and irritant side effects while their bacterial resistance was superior to chitosan, honey, and gelatin when used separately (Wang et al. 2012).

2.6. Ocular Tissue Engineering

Gelatin-based materials have been most successful in ocular tissue engineering as cell sheet carriers, with effective delivery of both corneal endothelial sheets to the posterior cornea (Lai et al. 20130, and also RPE (Retinal pigment epithelium) sheets to the sub-retinal space (Silverman and Hughes1989). Gelatin offers an excellent, low-cost starting substrate. Crosslinked gelatin scaffolds make up a small but important part of the ocular tissue engineering. If crosslinked using appropriate methods it could provide lower antigenic and immunogenic risk than its parent material. Gelatin and its derivatives have been used as potential scaffolds for corneal epithelium (Wang et al. 2012), corneal endothelium (de la Mata et al. 2013) and retinal pigment epithelium (Lai 2013), as a bio-artificial corneal stroma

(Lai 2013) and as a potential bio-adhesive in treatment of retinal detachment (Yamamoto et al. 2013). The range of crosslinking options used to strengthen gelatin scaffolds in this field. There is good evidence to suggest that cross-linkers may be preferable in terms of both cell compatibility and biocompatibility (Lai and Li 2010). Whilst there may be uses for glutaraldehyde to crosslink matrices, such as fragile electrospun matrices which are short-lived in aqueous solutions (Sisson et al. 2009), the risk of cell toxicity of excipients could be a potential issue. Gelatin methacrylamide offers a gel-based system with tunable matrix stiffness, which can be controlled without significantly changing the chemical composition, this material would be an effective tool in determining the optimum material properties for application in ocular tissue engineering. The utility of dehydrated gelatin discs in ocular tissue engineering has been dominated by application as a cell sheet carrier in the delivery of either endothelial cell sheets to the posterior cornea (Hsu et al. 2013), or retinal pigment epithelial cells to the sub-retinal space (Lai et al. 2013; Rose et al. 2014). The application of photo cross-linkable gelatin in corneal stromal tissue engineering is also foreseen.

CONCLUSION

Among the natural polymeric materials, gelatin offers great practical potential as a composite material in the biomedical field. The resulting gelatin-based materials from various processing techniques exhibit excellent biocompatibility, biodegradability, and porous structure. Gelatin has been developed in different forms including films/foams, porous scaffolds, and hydrogels. So far, there has been significant progress in tuning the physical and chemical properties of gelatin through changing the crosslinking process and blending it with other natural and synthetic biomaterials for specific applications. Gelatin blends with other polymers always produce high efficacy matrices with improved biomechanical and bio-affinity of the scaffolds.

REFERENCES

Abrams, D., Huang, Y., McQuarrie, S., Roa, W., Chen, H., Löbenberg, R., Azarmi, S., Miller, G. G. & Finlay, W. H. (2006). "Optimization of a two-step desolvation method for preparing gelatin nanoparticles and cell uptake studies in 143B osteosarcoma cancer cells" *Journal of Pharma and Pharmaceutical sciences*, 9, 124-32.

Ayvazyan, A., Morimoto, N., Kanda, N., Takemoto, S., Kawai, K., Sakamoto, Y., Taira, T. & Suzuki, S. (2011). "Collagen-gelatin scaffold impregnated with bFGF accelerates palatal wound healing of palatal mucosa in dogs". *Journal of Surgical Research*, 171, e247-e257.

Azimi, B., Nourpanah, P., Rabiee, M. & Arbab, S. (2014). "Producing gelatin nanoparticles as delivery system for bovine serum albumin" *Iranian biomedical journal*, 18, 34-40.

Balakrishnan, B., Mohanty, M., Umashankar, P. R. & Jayakrishnan, A. (2005). "Evaluation of an *in situ* forming hydrogel wound dressing based on oxidized alginate and gelatin" *Biomaterials*, 26, 6335-6342.

Barnett, S. E. & Irving, S. J. (1991). "Studies of wound healing and the effect of dressings" *High performance biomaterials*, 583-620.

Bose, S., Roy, M. & Bandyopadhyay, A. (2012). "Recent advances in bone tissue engineering scaffolds" *Trends in biotechnology*, 30, 546-554.

Burke, C. J., Hsu, T. A. & Volkin, D. B. (1999). "Formulation, stability, and delivery of live attenuated vaccines for human use" *Critical Reviews in Therapeutic Drug Carrier Systems*, 16(1).

Chen, Y. C., Lin, R. Z., Qi, H., Yang, Y., Bae, H., Melero-Martin, J. M. & Khademhosseini, A. (2012). "Functional human vascular network generated in photo crosslinkable gelatin methacrylate hydrogels" *Advanced functional materials*, 22, 2027-2039.

Cheng, Y. H., Hung, K. H., Tsai, T. H., Lee, C. J., Ku, R. Y., Chiu, A. W. H., Chiou, S. H. & Liu, C. J. L. (2014). "Sustained delivery of latanoprost by thermosensitive chitosan–gelatin-based hydrogel for controlling ocular hypertension" *Acta biomaterialia*, 10, 4360-4366.

Choi, Y. S., Hong, S. R., Lee, Y. M., Song, K. W., Park, M. H. & Nam, Y. S. (1999). "Studies on gelatin-containing artificial skin: II. Preparation and characterization of cross-linked gelatin-hyaluronate sponge". *Journal of Biomedical Materials Research: An Official Journal of The Society for Biomaterials, The Japanese Society for Biomaterials, and The Australian Society for Biomaterials and the Korean Society for Biomaterials*, *48*, 631-639.

Cui, L., Jia, J., Guo, Y., Liu, Y. & Zhu, P. (2014). "Preparation and characterization of IPN hydrogels composed of chitosan and gelatin cross-linked by genipin" *Carbohydrate polymers*, *99*, 31-38.

de la Mata, A., Nieto-Miguel, T., López-Paniagua, M., Galindo, S., Aguilar, M. R., García-Fernández, L., Gonzalo, S., Vázquez, B., San Román, J., Corrales, R. M. & Calonge, M. (2013). "Chitosan–gelatin biopolymers as carrier substrata for limbal epithelial stem cells" *Journal of Materials Science: Materials in Medicine*, *24*, 2819-2829.

Di Silvio, L. & Bonfield, W. (1999). "Biodegradable drug delivery system for the treatment of bone infection and repair" *Journal of Materials Science: Materials in Medicine*, *10*(10-11), 653-658.

Draye, J. P., Delaey, B., Van de Voorde, A., Van Den Bulcke, A., De Reu, B. & Schacht, E. (1998). "*In vitro* and *in vivo* biocompatibility of dextran dialdehyde cross-linked gelatin hydrogel films" *Biomaterials*, *19*, 1677-1687.

Duan, H., Feng, B., Guo, X., Wang, J., Zhao, L., Zhou, G., Liu, W., Cao, Y. & Zhang, W. J. (2013). "Engineering of epidermis skin grafts using electrospunnanofibrous gelatin/polycaprolactone membranes" *International journal of nanomedicine*, *8*, 2077-2084.

Enrione, J., Díaz-Calderón, P., Weinstein-Oppenheimer, C. R., Sánchez, E., Fuentes, M. A., Brown, D. I., Herrera, H. & Acevedo, C. A. (2013). "Designing a gelatin/chitosan/hyaluronic acid biopolymer using a thermophysical approach for use in tissue engineering" *Bioprocess and biosystems engineering*, *36*, 1947-1956.

Foox, M. & Zilberman, M. (2015). "Drug delivery from gelatin-based systems" *Expert opinion on drug delivery*, *12*, 1547-1563.

Gao, M., Liu, N., Li, Z., Wang, W., Li, C., Zhang, H., Chen, Y., Yu, Z. & Huang, Y. (2014). "A gelatin-based sol–gel procedure to synthesize the

LiFePO4/C nanocomposite for lithium ion batteries" *Solid State Ionics*, *258*, 8-12.

Gautam, S., Chou, C. F., Dinda, A. K., Potdar, P. D. & Mishra, N. C. (2014). "Surface modification of nanofibrouspolycaprolactone/gelatin composite scaffold by collagen type I grafting for skin tissue engineering" *Materials Science and Engineering: C*, *34*, 402-409.

Han, J., Lazarovici, P., Pomerantz, C., Chen, X., Wei, Y. & Lelkes, P. I. (2010). "Co-electrospun blends of PLGA, gelatin, and elastin as potential nonthrombogenic scaffolds for vascular tissue engineering" *Biomacromolecules*, *12*, 399-408.

Hanani, Z. N., Roos, Y. H. & Kerry, J. P. (2014). "Use and application of gelatin as potential biodegradable packaging materials for food products" *International journal of biological macromolecules*, *71*, 94-102.

Hench, L. & Jones, J. eds. (2005). "Biomaterials, artificial organs and tissue engineering". Elsevier.

Hoque, M. E., Nuge, T., Yeow, T. K., Nordin, N. & Prasad, R. G. S. V. (2015). "Gelatin based scaffolds for tissue engineering-a review" *Polymers Research Journal*, *9*, 15-32.

Hsu, W. M., Chen, K. H., Lai, J. Y. & Hsiue, G. H. (2013). "Transplantation of human corneal endothelial cells using functional biomaterials: poly (N-isopropylacrylamide) and gelatin" *Journal of Experimental & Clinical Medicine*, *5*, 56-64.

Ifkovits, J. L., Devlin, J. J., Eng, G., Martens, T. P., Vunjak-Novakovic, G. & Burdick, J. A. (2009). "Biodegradable fibrous scaffolds with tunable properties formed from photo-cross-linkable poly (glycerol sebacate)" *ACS applied materials & interfaces*, 1, 1878-1886.

Jaipan, P., Nguyen, A. & Narayan, R. J. (2017). "Gelatin-based hydrogels for biomedical applications" *MRS Communications*, *7*, 416-426.

Karim, A. A. & Bhat, R. (2009). "Fish gelatin: properties, challenges, and prospects as an alternative to mammalian gelatins" *Food hydrocolloids*, *23*, 563-576.

Kempen, D. H., Lu, L., Heijink, A., Hefferan, T. E., Creemers, L. B., Maran, A., Yaszemski, M. J. & Dhert, W. J. (2009). "Effect of local sequential

VEGF and BMP-2 delivery on ectopic and orthotopic bone regeneration" *Biomaterials, 30*(14), 2816-2825.

Khan, S. A. (2014). Gelatin Nanoparticles as Potential Nanocarriers for Macromolecular Drugs (Doctoral Dissertation, Philipps-University Marburg).

Kharaziha, M., Nikkhah, M., Shin, S. R., Annabi, N., Masoumi, N., Gaharwar, A. K., Camci-Unal, G. & Khademhosseini, A. (2013). "PGS: Gelatin nanofibrous scaffolds with tunable mechanical and structural properties for engineering cardiac tissues" *Biomaterials, 34*(27), 6355-6366.

Kim, S. W., Ogawa, T., Tabata, Y. & Nishimura, I. (2004). "Efficacy and cytotoxicity of cationic-agent–mediated nonviral gene transfer into osteoblasts" *Journal of Biomedical Materials Research Part A: An Official Journal of The Society for Biomaterials, The Japanese Society for Biomaterials, and The Australian Society for Biomaterials and the Korean Society for Biomaterials, 71*(2), 308-315.

Kuijpers, A. J., Engbers, G. H., van Wachem, P. B., Krijgsveld, J., Zaat, S. A., Dankert, J. & Feijen, J. (1998). "Controlled delivery of antibacterial proteins from biodegradable matrices" *Journal of controlled release, 53*(1-3), 235-247.

Lai, J. Y. & Li, Y. T. (2010). "Evaluation of cross-linked gelatin membranes as delivery carriers for retinal sheets" *Materials Science and Engineering: C, 30*(5), 677-685.

Lai, J. Y. (2013). "Corneal stromal cell growth on gelatin/chondroitin sulfate scaffolds modified at different NHS/EDC molar ratios" *International journal of molecular sciences, 14*(1), 2036-2055.

Lai, J. Y. (2013). "Influence of solvent composition on the performance of carbodiimide cross-linked gelatin carriers for retinal sheet delivery" *Journal of Materials Science: Materials in Medicine, 24*(9), 2201-2210.

Lai, J. Y., Ma, D. H. K., Lai, M. H., Li, Y. T., Chang, R. J. & Chen, L. M. (2013). "Characterization of cross-linked porous gelatin carriers and their interaction with corneal endothelium: biopolymer concentration effect" *PLoS One, 8*(1), e54058.

Lee, S. B., Kim, Y. H., Chong, M. S., Hong, S. H. & Lee, Y. M. (2005). "Study of gelatin-containing artificial skin V: fabrication of gelatin scaffolds using a salt-leaching method" *Biomaterials*, *26*, 1961-1968.

Li, J. H., Miao, J., Wu, J. L., Chen, S. F. & Zhang, Q. Q. (2014). "Preparation and characterization of active gelatin-based films incorporated with natural antioxidants" *Food Hydrocolloids*, *37*, 166-173.

Li, R. K., Jia, Z. Q., Weisel, R. D., Mickle, D. A., Choi, A. & Yau, T. M. (1999). "Survival and function of bioengineered cardiac grafts" *Circulation*, *100*(suppl_2), II-63.

Li, R. K., Yau, T. M., Weisel, R. D., Mickle, D. A., Sakai, T., Choi, A. & Jia, Z. Q. (2000). "Construction of a bioengineered cardiac graft" *The Journal of thoracic and cardiovascular surgery*, *119*, 368-375.

Li, W. J., Shanti, R. M. & Tuan, R. S. (2007). "Electrospinning technology for nanofibrous scaffolds in tissue engineering" *Nanotechnologies for the Life Sciences*, onlinedoi.org/10.1002/9783527610419.ntls0097.

Mariod, A. A. & Fadul, H. (2013). "Gelatin, source, extraction and industrial applications" *Acta Scientiarum Polonorum Technologia Alimentaria*, *12*, 135-147.

Metcalfe, A. D. & Ferguson, M. W. (2006). "Tissue engineering of replacement skin: the crossroads of biomaterials, wound healing, embryonic development, stem cells and regeneration" *Journal of the Royal Society Interface*, *4*, 413-437.

Morimoto, N., Yoshimura, K., Niimi, M., Ito, T., Aya, R., Fujitaka, J., Tada, H., Teramukai, S., Murayama, T., Toyooka, C. & Miura, K. (2013). "Novel collagen/gelatin scaffold with sustained release of basic fibroblast growth factor: clinical trial for chronic skin ulcers" *Tissue Engineering Part A*, *19*, 1931-1940.

Nagiah, N., Madhavi, L., Anitha, R., Anandan, C., Srinivasan, N. T. & Sivagnanam, U. T. (2013). "Development and characterization of coaxially electrospun gelatin coated poly (3-hydroxybutyric acid) thin films as potential scaffolds for skin regeneration" *Materials Science and Engineering: C*, *33*, 4444-4452.

Nerurkar, N. L., Elliott, D. M. & Mauck, R. L. (2007). "Mechanics of oriented electrospunnanofibrous scaffolds for annulus fibrosus tissue engineering" *Journal of orthopaedic research, 25*, 1018-1028.

Nikkhah, M., Eshak, N., Zorlutuna, P., Annabi, N., Castello, M., Kim, K., Dolatshahi-Pirouz, A., Edalat, F., Bae, H., Yang, Y. & Khademhosseini, A. (2012). "Directed endothelial cell morphogenesis in micropatterned gelatin methacrylate hydrogels" *Biomaterials, 33*, 9009-9018.

Ninan, G., Jose, J. & Abubacker, Z. (2011). "Preparation and characterization of gelatin extracted from the skins of rohu (Labeorohita) and common carp (Cyprinuscarpio)" *Journal of Food Processing and Preservation, 35*, 143-162.

Ozawa, T., Mickle, D. A., Weisel, R. D., Matsubayashi, K., Fujii, T., Fedak, P. W., Koyama, N., Ikada, Y. & Li, R. K. (2004). "Tissue-engineered grafts matured in the right ventricular outflow tract" *Cell transplantation, 13*, 169-177.

Panduranga Rao, K. (1996). "Recent developments of collagen-based materials for medical applications and drug delivery systems" *Journal of Biomaterials Science*, Polymer Edition, *7*, 623-645.

Parke, N. G. & Povey, M. J. W. (2012). "Ultrasonic study of the gelation of gelatin: phase diagram, hysteresis and kinetics" *Food Hydrocolloids, 26*, 99-107.

Patel, Z. S., Yamamoto, M., Ueda, H., Tabata, Y. & Mikos, A. G. (2008). "Biodegradable gelatin microparticles as delivery systems for the controlled release of bone morphogenetic protein-2" *Acta biomaterialia, 4*, 1126-1138.

Patel, Z. S., Young, S., Tabata, Y., Jansen, J. A., Wong, M. E. & Mikos, A. G. (2008). "Dual delivery of an angiogenic and an osteogenic growth factor for bone regeneration in a critical size defect model" *Bone, 43*, 931-940.

Pereira, I. H., Ayres, E., Averous, L., Schlatter, G., Hebraud, A., de Paula, A. C. C., Viana, P. H. L., Goes, A. M. & Oréfice, R. L. (2014). "Differentiation of human adipose-derived stem cells seeded on mineralized electrospun co-axial poly (ε-caprolactone)(PCL)/gelatin nanofibers" *Journal of Materials Science: Materials in Medicine*, *25*, 1137-1148.

Perng, C. K., Kao, C. L., Yang, Y. P., Lin, H. T., Lin, W. B., Chu, Y. R., Wang, H. J., Ma, H., Ku, H. H. & Chiou, S. H. (2008). "Culturing adult human bone marrow stem cells on gelatin scaffold with pNIPAAm as transplanted grafts for skin regeneration" *Journal of Biomedical Materials Research Part A: An Official Journal of The Society for Biomaterials, The Japanese Society for Biomaterials, and The Australian Society for Biomaterials and the Korean Society for Biomaterials*, *84*, 622-630.

Pollack, S. V. (1990). "Silicone, fibrel, and collagen implantation for facial lines and wrinkles" *The Journal of dermatologic surgery and oncology*, *16*, 957-961.

Powell, H. M. & Boyce, S. T. (2008). "Fiber density of electrospun gelatin scaffolds regulates morphogenesis of dermal–epidermal skin substitutes" *Journal of Biomedical Materials Research Part A: An Official Journal of The Society for Biomaterials, The Japanese Society for Biomaterials, and The Australian Society for Biomaterials and the Korean Society for Biomaterials*, *84*, 1078-1086.

Prata, A. S. & Grosso, C. R. F. (2015). "Production of microparticles with gelatin and chitosan" *Carbohydrate polymers*, *116*, 292-299.

Rajan, M. & Raj, V. (2013). "Formation and characterization of chitosan-polylacticacid-polyethylene glycol-gelatin nanoparticles: A novel biosystem for controlled drug delivery" *Carbohydrate polymers*, *98*, 951-958.

Rane, A. A. & Christman, K. L. (2011). "Biomaterials for the treatment of myocardial infarction: a 5-year update" *Journal of the American College of Cardiology*, *58*, 2615-2629.

Rose, J., Pacelli, S., Haj, A., Dua, H., Hopkinson, A., White, L. & Rose, F. (2014). "Gelatin-based materials in ocular tissue engineering" *Materials*, *7*, 3106-313.

Saddler, J. M. & Horsey, P. J. (1987). "The new generation gelatins: a review of their history, manufacture and properties" *Anaesthesia*, *42*, 998-1004.

Santoro, M., Tatara, A. M. & Mikos, A. G. (2014). "Gelatin carriers for drug and cell delivery in tissue engineering" *Journal of controlled release*, *190*, 210-218.

Schrieber, R. & Gareis, H. (2007). "Gelatine handbook: theory and industrial practice" John Wiley & Sons.

Silverman, M. S. & Hughes, S. E. (1989). "Transplantation of photoreceptors to light-damaged retina" *Investigative ophthalmology & visual science*, *30*, 1684-1690.

Sisson, K., Zhang, C., Farach-Carson, M. C., Chase, D. B. & Rabolt, J. F. (2009). "Evaluation of cross-linking methods for electrospun gelatin on cell growth and viability" *Biomacromolecules*, *10*, 1675-1680.

Su, K. & Wang, C. (2015). "Recent advances in the use of gelatin in biomedical research" *Biotechnology letters*, *37*, 2139-2145.

Tamayol, A., Akbari, M., Annabi, N., Paul, A., Khademhosseini, A. & Juncker, D. (2013). "Fiber-based tissue engineering: progress, challenges, and opportunities" *Biotechnology advances*, *31*, 669-687.

Tanaka, F. (2003). "Thermoreversible gelation driven by coil-to-helix transition of polymers" *Macromolecules*, *36*, 5392-5405.

Tang, G., Zhang, H., Zhao, Y., Zhang, Y., Li, X. & Yuan, X. (2012). "Preparation of PLGA scaffolds with graded pores by using a gelatin-microsphere template as porogen" *Journal of Biomaterials Science, Polymer Edition*, *23*, 2241-2257.

Vatankhah, E., Prabhakaran, M. P., Jin, G., Mobarakeh, L. G. & Ramakrishna, S. (2014). "Development of nanofibrous cellulose acetate/gelatin skin substitutes for variety wound treatment applications" *Journal of biomaterials applications*, *28*, 909-921.

Wang, H., Boerman, O. C., Sariibrahimoglu, K., Li, Y., Jansen, J. A. & Leeuwenburgh, S. C. (2012). "Comparison of micro-vs. Nano-structured colloidal gelatin gels for sustained delivery of osteogenic proteins: Bone morphogenetic protein-2 and alkaline phosphatase" *Biomaterials*, *33*, 8695-8703.

Wang, T., Zhu, X. K., Xue, X. T. & Wu, D. Y. (2012). "Hydrogel sheets of chitosan, honey and gelatin as burn wound dressings" *Carbohydrate polymers*, *88*, 75-83.

Wen, Y., Jiang, B., Cui, J., Li, G., Yu, M., Wang, F., Zhang, G., Nan, X., Yue, W., Xu, X. & Pei, X. (2013). "Superior osteogenic capacity of different mesenchymal stem cells for bone tissue engineering" *Oral surgery, oral medicine, oral pathology and oral radiology*, *116*(5), e324-e332.

Winter, G. D. (1962). "Formation of the scab and the rate of epithelization of superficial wounds in the skin of the young domestic pig" *Nature*, *193*, 293-294.

Yaffe, A., Herman, A., Bahar, H. & Binderman, I. (2003). "Combined local application of tetracycline and bisphosphonate reduces alveolar bone resorption in rats" *Journal of periodontology*, *74*, 1038-1042.

Yamamoto, S., Hirata, A., Ishikawa, S., Ohta, K., Nakamura, K. I. & Okinami, S. (2013). "Feasibility of using gelatin-microbial transglutaminase complex to repair experimental retinal detachment in rabbit eyes" *Graefe's Archive for Clinical and Experimental Ophthalmology*, *251*, 1109-1114.

Zhang, Y. Z., Venugopal, J., Huang, Z. M., Lim, C. T. & Ramakrishna, S. 2006 "Crosslinking of the electrospun gelatin nanofibers" *Polymer*, *47*, 2911-2917.

In: Biocomposites in Bio-Medicine
Editors: Mudasir Ahmad et al.

ISBN: 978-1-53616-247-9
© 2019 Nova Science Publishers, Inc.

Chapter 4

POLYLACTIDE (PLA) BASED NANOCOMPOSITES FOR APPLICATIONS IN ANTIBACTERIAL/MICROBIAL AND BIOMEDICAL ENGINEERING

Sapana Jadoun[*]
School of Basic & Applied Sciences, Department of Chemistry,
Lingayas Vidyapeeth, Faridabad, Haryana, India

ABSTRACT

For the last few decades, there has been growing interest in bio-based polymers and nanocomposites open an opportunity for the use of new, high-performance material. The use of biodegradable polymers and nanocomposites are of great importance currently in many applications, Polylactide (PLA) represents the best polymeric substitutes in the framework of environmentally friendly and sustainable processes and products for several petropolymers due to its renewability, biocompatibility, ease of surface chemistry modification, biodegradability, good thermomechanical and optical properties. Having the above properties polylactide (PLA) nanocomposite shows immense potential in food packaging, antimicrobial as well as in pharmacology and biomedical engineering areas.

Keywords: polylactide (PLA), nanocomposites, food packaging, biomedicine

INTRODUCTION

Polylactide (PLA) is a thermoplastic that can be derived from renewable sources and degrades to nontoxic compounds in landfills (Martin and Averous 2001; Tsuji and Ikada 1998). Polylactide (PLA) has been the leader in all biopolymers due to its outstanding mechanical properties, biodegradability, renewability, and relatively low cost and also justify environmental concerns of greenhouse gas emissions, environmental pollution and the depletion of fossil resource (Auras, Harte, and Selke 2004; Kümmerer 2007; Jenck, Agterberg, and Droescher 2004). It is a polymer of monomer lactic acid, which may be easily produced by carbohydrate feedstock's fermentation. Hence, PLA provides more disposal options and its production is less environmentally burdensome in comparison to other traditional petroleum-based plastics (Doi and Steinbüchel 2002; Lunt 1998). Low molecular weight PLA was firstly prepared by *Pelouze* in 1845 by the action of condensation of l-lactic acid followed by removing of water continuously (Carothers, Dorough, and Natta 1932). To substitute the conventional petroleum-based plastics, Polylactic acid (PLA) has been explored recently by researchers or polymer scientists as potential biopolymer (Sinha Ray, Maiti, et al. 2002; Sinha Ray et al. 2003; Ray and Okamoto 2003). PLA, in comparison to some other polymers, is stiff and brittle with low impact strength and low deformation at break (Jacobsen et al. 1999). In recent, PLA has grabbed attention as of biodegradable polymers, though, as packaging material, the use of PLA is still a barrier due to its high cost and low performance as compared to other commodity polymers. The most important limitation is its low gas barrier properties for the application of PLA in food packaging. For applications in various fields, PLA suffers some other limitations like heat distortion temperature, low thermal resistance, and rate of crystallization, while some other precise properties are essential by different end-use sectors such as antistatic to conductive electrical characteristics, flame retardancy, antibacterial, anti-UV or barrier properties, etc.

Polymer nanocomposites have grabbed a lot of attention from the last few years. These are low cost and high-performance materials for applications in various fields from tissue engineering to automotive to food packaging have become enchanting to researchers around the world (Vaia and Giannelis 2001; Alexandre and Dubois 2000; Giannelis 1996). Nanocomposites technology has the great potential to enhance polymer properties and inflate the applications of PLA, therefore, by adding nanofillers in PLA represents an interesting way to outspread and to enhance the properties of PLA (Raquez et al. 2013; Thellen et al. 2005; Rhim, Hong, and Ha 2009; Sinclair 1996). A number of researchers have been worked on PLA-based nanocomposites with layered silicates so as to mark highly exfoliated structures. *Bordes* et al. (Bordes, Pollet, and Avérous 2009) reported routes for the synthesis of PLA/layered silicate nanocomposites which was based on solvent intercalation, melt-intercalation and in situ intercalation.

METHODS

Preparation and Properties of Polylactide (PLA) Nanocomposites

Sinha Ray and Maiti (2002) synthesized polylactide (PLA)/layered silicate nanocomposites by simple melt extrusion of PLA with organically modified montmorillonite. These intercalated nanocomposites revealed outstanding enhancement of materials properties in both melt and solid states in comparison to PLA matrices without clay. Cabedo (2006) reported nanocomposites of amorphous PLA and chemically modified kaolinite and noticed good interaction within polymer and clay led to an increase in oxygen barrier properties of about 50%. They also studied the addition of plasticizers to conquer the inherent brittleness of PLA. Schmidt, Shah, and Giannelis (2002) developed many poly(l-lactic acid) (PLA) nanocomposites which were based on different layered inorganics. These nanocomposites exhibited enhanced mechanical properties with higher moduli in compare to pure PLA. The increment was above T_g, by which work temperature was enhanced and this enhancement did not hinder biodegradation. In nanocomposites, the rate of biodegradation was enhanced six to ten times and it was cleared by marine respirometry and crystallinity measurements in solution pretending a physiological environment. PLA/PBAT bio-nano composites were prepared by *Moustafa* and coworkers for their application in antimicrobial natural rosin for green packaging. They used green modification method of organoclay, non-toxic reinforcing material makes the material to maintain its green character. The attained results revealed the outstanding possibility of using expanded OC modified PLA/PBAT polymer blends in which green material antimicrobial natural rosin was added, for their applications in food packaging and biomembranes (Moustafa et al. 2017).

Table 1. Comparison of material properties between neat PLA and PLACN4 reprinted with permission from Nano Letters, 2002, 2 (10), pp 1093–1096. Copyright (2002) American Chemical Society

Material properties	Neat PLA	PLACN4
Storage modulus/GPa at 25°C	1.63	2.32
Flexural modulus/GPa at 25°C	4.8	5.5
Flexural strength/MPa at 25°C	86	134
Distortion at break/%	1.9	3.1
HDT/°C	76.2	94
O_2 gas permeability coefficient (mL.mm.m^{-2}.day^{-1}.MPa^{-1})	200	177

Ray and coworkers developed polylactide (PLA)-layered silicate nanocomposite and studied material properties and biodegradability. They found that material properties were increased after nanocomposite formation in comparison to neat PLA, Table 1 (Sinha Ray, Yamada, et al. 2002). D. R. Paul and Robeson (2008) reported that the addition of montmorillonite increased the biodegradation of PLA under compost. In these conditions, PLA firstly fragmented and followed by a biodegradation process, when PLA underwent fragmented to about 10,000 g/mol.

Sabet and Katbab (2009) prepared PLA based nanocomposites with improved biodegradability and abridged oxygen permeability via melt hybridization of poly (lactic acid) (PLA) and organomodified clay which showed a correlation between the structure of nanocomposites and rate of biodegradation.

Preparation of Poly(L-lactide)/layered aluminosilicate nanocomposites in the presence of two organo-modified montmorillonites by ring-opening polymerization was reported by Paul and coworkers (M. A. Paul et al. 2003). They suggested that the obtained exfoliated nanocomposites having enhanced thermal stability were attained by directly grafting of polymer chains on the surface of clay via hydroxyl-functionalized ammonium cations or these nanocomposites with high molecular weight were obtained via solid-state polymerization (Katiyar and Nanavati 2011). As sepiolite/PLA nanocomposites are less studied, the PLA nanocomposites melt-elaboration and characterization in the presence of Cloisite 30B and sepiolite was studied by Fukushima and coworkers (Fukushima, Tabuani, and Camino 2009).

Polylactide (PLA) nanocomposites were prepared by solution and melt mixing in the presence of carbon nanotubes (CNTs) for the studies of crystallization kinetics and morphology. Figure 1, represents the DSC cooling traces for nanocomposites cooled from the melt at various rates. Neat PLA showed very slow crystallization kinetics while with increasing CNT content faster crystallization kinetics are attained (Barrau et al. 2011).

Poly(lactic acid) (PLA) with organically modified montmorillonite (oMMT) in the presence of triallyl cyanurate (TAC), have been cross-linked by high-energy electrons in order to prepare its nanocomposites. TEM of PLA nanocomposites, Figure 2, revealed the internal structure of composites, like the dispersion position of the nanofiller in the matrix (Wang et al. 2012). Zheng (2009) prepared biocompatible (PDLLA)/magnetite (Fe_3O_4) nanocomposites by chemical co-precipitation and analysis of these were done by glass transition temperature (Tg), micro-surface morphology, mechanical properties, and functional groups change. Their shape memory effect was also reported in their studies.

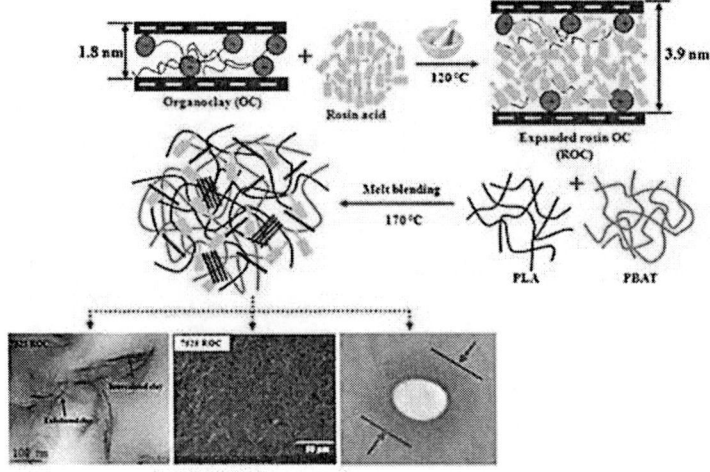

Figure 1. Synthetic scheme of PLA/PBAT/ROC bionanocomposite. Reprinted with permission from *ACS Appl. Mater. Interfaces, 2017, 9 (23), pp 20132–20141*. Copyright (2017) American Chemical Society.

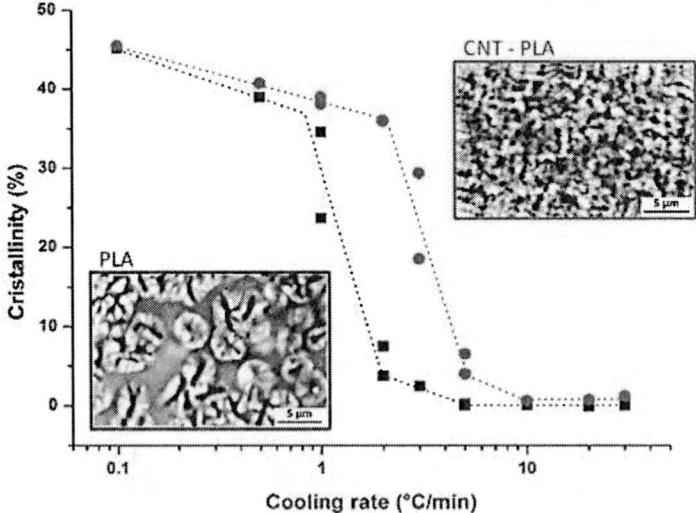

Figure 2. PLA crystal content versus cooling rate for NT0 (black squares), NT01 (green triangles), and NT1 (red circles). Reprinted with permission from *Macromolecules*, 2011, 44 (16), pp 6496–6502. Copyright (2011) American Chemical Society.

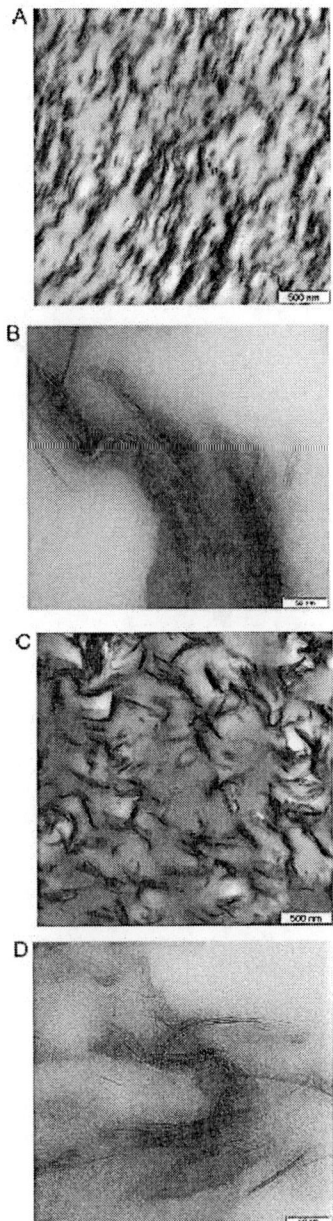

Figure 3. TEM patterns of PLA nanocomposites showing the nature of the dispersion of nanoclay in the matrix: (A, B) PLA-MMT-TAC 0kGy and (C, D) PLA-MMT-TAC 70kGy. Reprinted with permission from *Langmuir, 2012, 28 (34), pp 12601–12608*. Copyright (2012) American Chemical Society.

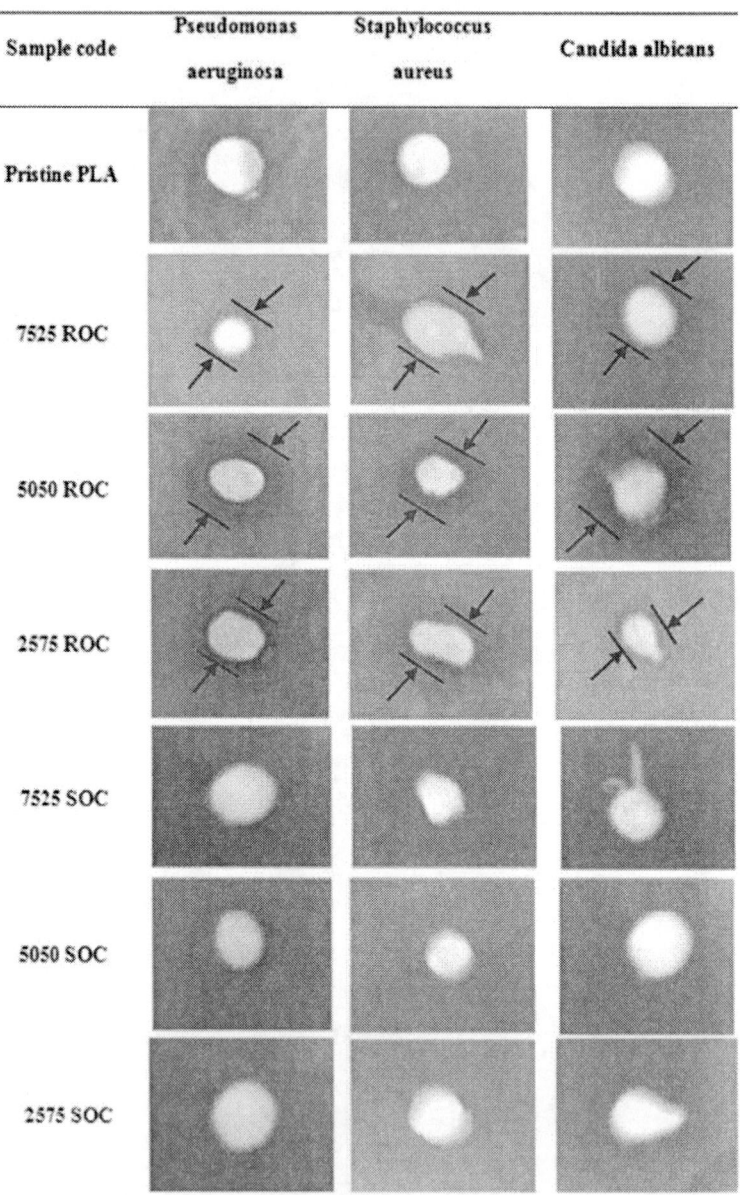

Figure 4. Antimicrobial activity for pristine PLA and its blends with different ratios of PBAT containing 2.5 w% of ROC or St. Acid against Pseudomonas Aeruginosa, Staphylococcus aureus, and Candida Albicans. Reprinted with permission from *ACS Appl. Mater. Interfaces, 2017, 9 (23), pp 20132–20141*. Copyright (2017) American Chemical Society.

Applications

As a biodegradable polymer, PLA has numerous applications in the biomedical field because of its biocompatibility features as well as good thermal plasticity, mechanical properties and is eagerly fabricated made it a promising polymer for several end-use application (Ray et al. 2003).

Biomedical

Kim, Lee, and Knowles (2006) developed PLA based nanocomposites in which in the suspension of biopolymer poly(lactic acid) (PLA) bioceramic hydroxyapatite (HA) was kept with the aim to insert a surfactant hydroxystearic acid (HSA) between the hydrophobic chloroform-dissolved PLA and hydrophilic HA powder. These nanocomposites were found useful in tissue engineering applications, mainly as three-dimensional substrates for bone growth. Nanocomposites of PLA was prepared by accumulating anticancer drug daunorubicin on PLA nanofibers and TiO_2 nanoparticles combination. Studies suggested that the above drug molecule is easily assembled in nanocomposites surface and can enable the drug infiltration and buildup on the target leukemia K562 cells. These nanocomposites having ease of surface chemistry modification, good biocompatibility, and very high surface area makes it a suitable candidate for biomedical engineering areas and pharmacology (Chen et al. 2007). Boccaccini (2010) reviewed various nanocomposites including poly(lactic acid) and suggested their mechanical, physicochemical and biological properties of introducing nanoscale bioactive in that type of biodegradable nanocomposites and revealed the chances of these materials in biomedical applications. Nanocomposites of polylactic acid/starch/poly ε-caprolactone (PLASCL20) were prepared via melt blending by mixing abovesaid with nanohydroxyapatite (nHA). The addition of 3% nHA in these nanocomposites enhanced the hydrophilicity, antibacterial activity, hydrolytic degradation, and the drug release as compare to PLASCL20. These were found suitable as antibacterial contenders for several medical applications along with the least side effects because of the controlled release of triclosan (Davachi et al. 2017).

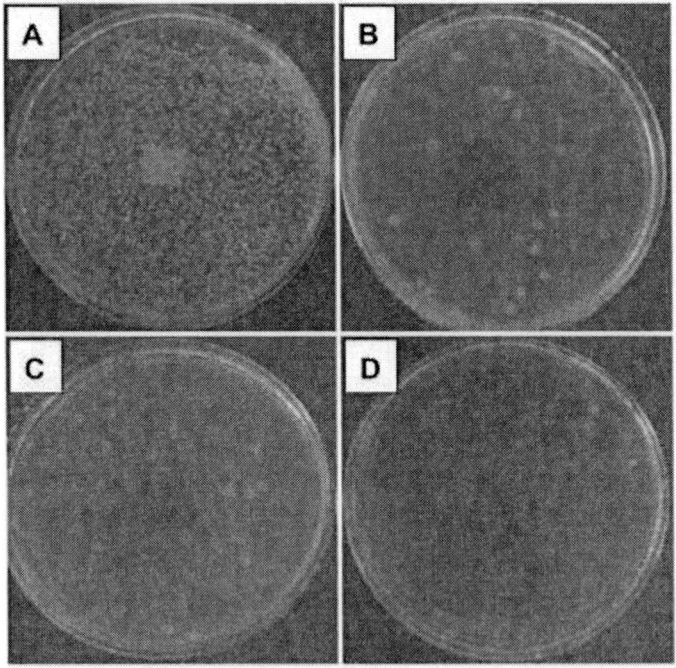

Figure 5. Comparison of inhibition zone test for Vibrio parahaemolyticus between PLA (A), Ag/PLA-NC content 8 (B), 16 (C), and 32 (D) wt% respectively.

The development of silver/poly (lactic acid) nanocomposite (Ag/PLA-NC) films was done by *Shameli* and his coworkers. They investigated that silver nanoparticles were synthesized via chemical reduction method into biodegradable PLA in diphase solvent in which sodium borohydride was used as a reducing agent. Silver nitrate acted as a polymeric matrix and sodium borohydride acted as a precursor in the PLA nanocomposite preparation. Ag/PLA-NC films revealed antibacterial activity, Figure 5, against Gram-positive bacteria (Staphylococcus aureus) and Gram-negative bacteria (Escherichia coli and Vibrio parahaemolyticus) by diffusion method using Muller–Hinton agar and the results revealed that these films can be used as an antibacterial scaffold for medical application and tissue engineering (Shameli et al. 2010). Nieddu (2009) reported PLA nanocomposites with different layered silicates nanoclays like fluorohectorites and montmorillonites with or without organic modifiers for their application in biodegradation in blood plasma. Development of sol-gel bioactive glass/poly(l-lactide) nanocomposite scaffolds were reported by *El-Kady* and coworkers. In vitro bioactivity studies of these were found potentially applicable in bone engineering (El-Kady, Ali, and Farag 2010).

Others

Nanocomposite composed by PLA and montmorillonite layered silicate may lead to barrier properties suitable for food packaging applications (Thellen et al. 2005). In the chain, Rhim, Park, and Ha (2013) reported the applications of PLA nanocomposites in food packaging as these nanocomposites to have the potential of improvement of packaging performance as well as their biodegradability, mechanical, thermal and antimicrobial properties are perfect for the food packaging. PLA/Cloisite 30B composite film films were prepared for the improvement in their tensile strength, water vapor barrier, and antimicrobial properties. Tensile strength, elongation at break and water vapor permeability of nanocomposites were found $3.0 \pm 0.1\%$ and 1.8×10^{-11} gm/m² s Pa respectively and bacteriostatic function against *Listeria monocytogenes* (Rhim, Hong, and Ha 2009). The nanocomposite of PLA and montmorillonite-layered silicate was found useful in food packaging material due to its good barrier properties (Shibata et al. 2006). Sinha Ray and coworkers reviewed recent developments and properties of nanocomposites including PLA (Ray and Bousmina 2005). Studies of photodegradation of PLA-TiO_2 nanocomposites under UV light was done by *Nakayama* and coworkers and suggested that nanocomposites photo degradability can be efficiently promoted and their application in food packaging (Nakayama and Hayashi 2007).

CONCLUSION

The evolution of layered silicate-based PLA nanocomposites fruitfully created a sustainable material with improved thermal, physical, and chemical properties, to be an alternative to petroleum-based materials. Primarily, most of its applications were limited to short-time uses like the packaging but now it is expanded to the biomedical sector due to its biodegradable property. Fascinatingly, due to the reduction of petroleum resources, PLA is now perceiving more and more attention as a valuable sourced polymer alternative in longstanding applications like electronics and automotive. Hence, the present chapter highlights the main developments and researches in PLA-based nanocomposites during this last decade.

REFERENCES

Alexandre, Michael, and Philippe Dubois. 2000. "Polymer-Layered Silicate Nanocomposites: Preparation, Properties and Uses of a New Class of Materials." *Materials Science and Engineering: R: Reports* 28 (1–2). Elsevier: 1–63.

Auras, Rafael, Bruce Harte, and Susan Selke. 2004. "An Overview of Polylactides as Packaging Materials." *Macromolecular Bioscience* 4 (9). John Wiley & Sons, Ltd: 835–64. doi:10.1002/mabi.200400043.

Barrau, S, C Vanmansart, M Moreau, A Addad, G Stoclet, J.-M. Lefebvre, and R Seguela. 2011. "Crystallization Behavior of Carbon Nanotube−Polylactide Nanocomposites." *Macromolecules* 44 (16). American Chemical Society: 6496–6502. doi:10.1021/ma200842n.

Boccaccini, Aldo R, Melek Erol, Wendelin J Stark, Dirk Mohn, Zhongkui Hong, and João F Mano. 2010. "Polymer/Bioactive Glass Nanocomposites for Biomedical Applications: A Review." *Composites Science and Technology* 70 (13): 1764–76. doi: https://doi.org/10.1016/j.compscitech.2010.06.002.

Bordes, Perrine, Eric Pollet, and Luc Avérous. 2009. "Nano-Biocomposites: Biodegradable Polyester/Nanoclay Systems." *Progress in Polymer Science* 34 (2): 125–55. doi: https://doi.org/10.1016/j.progpolymsci.2008.10.002.

Cabedo, Lluís, José Luis Feijoo, María Pilar Villanueva, José María Lagarón, and Enrique Giménez. 2006. "Optimization of Biodegradable Nanocomposites Based on APLA/PCL Blends for Food Packaging

Applications." In *Macromolecular Symposia*, 233:191–97. Wiley Online Library.

Carothers, Wallace H, G L Dorough, and F J van Natta. 1932. "Studies Of Polymerization and Ring Formation. X. The Reversible Polymerization of Six-Membered Cyclic Esters." *Journal of the American Chemical Society* 54 (2). American Chemical Society: 761–72. doi:10.102 1/ja01341a046.

Chen, Chen, Gang Lv, Chao Pan, Min Song, Chunhui Wu, Dadong Guo, Xuemei Wang, Baoan Chen, and Zhongze Gu. 2007. "Poly(Lactic Acid) (PLA) Based Nanocomposites—a Novel Way of Drug-Releasing." *Biomedical Materials* 2 (4). IOP Publishing: L1–4. doi:10.1088/1748-6041/2/4/l01.

Davachi, Seyed Mohammad, Behzad Shiroud Heidari, Iman Hejazi, Javad Seyfi, Erfan Oliaei, Arman Farzaneh, and Hamid Rashedi. 2017. "Interface Modified Polylactic Acid/Starch/Poly ε-Caprolactone Antibacterial Nanocomposite Blends for Medical Applications." *Carbohydrate Polymers* 155: 336–44. doi: https://doi.org/10.1016/j.carbpol.2016.08.037.

Doi, Yoshiharu, and Alexander Steinbüchel. 2002. *Biopolymers, Polyesters III-Applications and Commercial Products*. Vol. 4. Wiley-Blackwell.

El-Kady, Abeer M, Ashraf F Ali, and Mohmmad M Farag. 2010. "Development, Characterization, and in Vitro Bioactivity Studies of Sol–gel Bioactive Glass/Poly(l-Lactide) Nanocomposite Scaffolds." *Materials Science and Engineering: C* 30 (1): 120–31. doi: https://doi.org/10.1016/j.msec.2009.09.008.

Fukushima, K, D Tabuani, and G Camino. 2009. "Nanocomposites of PLA and PCL Based on Montmorillonite and Sepiolite." *Materials Science and Engineering: C* 29 (4): 1433–41. doi: https://doi.org/10.1016/j.msec.2008.11.005.

Giannelis, Emmanuel P. 1996. "Polymer Layered Silicate Nanocomposites." *Advanced Materials* 8 (1). Wiley Online Library: 29–35.

Jacobsen, Sven, H G Fritz, Ph Degée, P H Dubois, and Robert Jérôme. 1999. "Polylactide (PLA)—a New Way of Production." *Polymer Engineering & Science* 39 (7). Wiley Online Library: 1311–19.

Jenck, Jean F, Frank Agterberg, and Michael J Droescher. 2004. "Products and Processes for a Sustainable Chemical Industry: A Review of Achievements and Prospects." *Green Chemistry* 6 (11). The Royal Society of Chemistry: 544–56. doi:10.1039/B406854H.

Katiyar, Vimal, and Hemant Nanavati. 2011. "High Molecular Weight Poly (L-Lactic Acid) Clay Nanocomposites via Solid-State Polymerization." *Polymer Composites* 32 (3). John Wiley & Sons, Ltd: 497–509. doi:10.1002/pc.21069.

Kim, Hae-Won, Hae-Hyoung Lee, and J C Knowles. 2006. "Electrospinning Biomedical Nanocomposite Fibers of Hydroxyapatite/Poly(Lactic Acid) for Bone Regeneration." *Journal of Biomedical Materials Research Part A* 79A (3). John Wiley & Sons, Ltd: 643–49. doi:10.1002/jbm.a.30866.

Kümmerer, Klaus. 2007. "Sustainable from the Very Beginning: Rational Design of Molecules by Life Cycle Engineering as an Important Approach for Green Pharmacy and Green Chemistry." *Green Chemistry* 9 (8). The Royal Society of Chemistry: 899–907. doi:10.1039/B618298B.

Lunt, James. 1998. "Large-Scale Production, Properties and Commercial Applications of Polylactic Acid Polymers." *Polymer Degradation and Stability* 59 (1–3). Elsevier: 145–52.

Martin, O, and L Averous. 2001. "Poly (Lactic Acid): Plasticization and Properties of Biodegradable Multiphase Systems." *Polymer* 42 (14). Elsevier: 6209–19.

Moustafa, Hesham, Nadia El Kissi, Ahmed I Abou-Kandil, Mohamed S Abdel-Aziz, and Alain Dufresne. 2017. "PLA/PBAT Bionanocomposites with Antimicrobial Natural Rosin for Green Packaging." *ACS Applied Materials & Interfaces* 9 (23). American Chemical Society: 20132–41. doi:10.1021/acsami.7b05557.

Nakayama, Norio, and Toyoharu Hayashi. 2007. "Preparation and Characterization of Poly (L-Lactic Acid)/TiO2 Nanoparticle

Nanocomposite Films with High Transparency and Efficient Photodegradability." *Polymer Degradation and Stability* 92 (7). Elsevier: 1255–64.

Nieddu, Erika, L Mazzucco, P Gentile, T Benko, V Balbo, R Mandrile, and G Ciardelli. 2009. "Preparation and Biodegradation of Clay Composites of PLA." *Reactive and Functional Polymers* 69 (6): 371–79. doi: https://doi.org/10.1016/j.reactfunctpolym.2009.03.002.

Paul, D R, and L M Robeson. 2008. "Polymer Nanotechnology: Nanocomposites." *Polymer* 49 (15): 3187–3204. doi: https://doi.org/10.1016/j.polymer.2008.04.017.

Paul, Marie-Amélie, Michaël Alexandre, Philippe Degée, Cédric Calberg, Robert Jérôme, and Philippe Dubois. 2003. "Exfoliated Polylactide/Clay Nanocomposites by In-Situ Coordination–Insertion Polymerization." *Macromolecular Rapid Communications* 24 (9). John Wiley & Sons, Ltd: 561–66. doi:10.1002/marc.200390082.

Raquez, Jean-Marie, Youssef Habibi, Marius Murariu, and Philippe Dubois. 2013. "Polylactide (PLA)-Based Nanocomposites." *Progress in Polymer Science* 38 (10): 1504–42. doi: https://doi.org/10.1016/j.progpolymsci.2013.05.014.

Ray, Suprakas Sinha, and Mosto Bousmina. 2005. "Biodegradable Polymers and Their Layered Silicate Nanocomposites: In Greening the 21st Century Materials World." *Progress in Materials Science* 50 (8). Elsevier: 962–1079.

Ray, Suprakas Sinha, and Masami Okamoto. 2003. "Polymer/Layered Silicate Nanocomposites: A Review from Preparation to Processing." *Progress in Polymer Science* 28 (11). Elsevier: 1539–1641.

Ray, Suprakas Sinha, Kazunobu Yamada, Masami Okamoto, Youhei Fujimoto, Akinobu Ogami, and Kazue Ueda. 2003. "New Polylactide/Layered Silicate Nanocomposites. 5. Designing of Materials with Desired Properties." *Polymer* 44 (21). Elsevier: 6633–46.

Rhim, Jong-Whan, Seok-In Hong, and Chang-Sik Ha. 2009. "Tensile, Water Vapor Barrier and Antimicrobial Properties of PLA/Nanoclay Composite Films." *LWT-Food Science and Technology* 42 (2). Elsevier: 612–17.

Rhim, Jong-Whan, Hwan-Man Park, and Chang-Sik Ha. 2013. "Bio-Nanocomposites for Food Packaging Applications." *Progress in Polymer Science* 38 (10): 1629–52. doi: https://doi.org/10.1016/j.progpolymsci.2013.05.008.

Sabet, S Shafiei, and A A Katbab. 2009. "Interfacially Compatibilized Poly(Lactic Acid) and Poly(Lactic Acid)/Polycaprolactone/Organoclay Nanocomposites with Improved Biodegradability and Barrier Properties: Effects of the Compatibilizer Structural Parameters and Feeding Route." *Journal of Applied Polymer Science* 111 (4). John Wiley & Sons, Ltd: 1954–63. doi:10.1002/app.29210.

Schmidt, Daniel, Deepak Shah, and Emmanuel P Giannelis. 2002. "New Advances in Polymer/Layered Silicate Nanocomposites." *Current Opinion in Solid State and Materials Science* 6 (3). Elsevier: 205–12.

Shameli, Kamyar, Mansor Bin Ahmad, Wan Md Zin Wan Yunus, Nor Azowa Ibrahim, Russly Abdul Rahman, Maryam Jokar, and Majid Darroudi. 2010. "Silver/Poly (Lactic Acid) Nanocomposites: Preparation, Characterization, and Antibacterial Activity." *International Journal of Nanomedicine* 5. Dove Press: 573.

Shibata, Mitsuhiro, Yoshihiro Someya, Masato Orihara, and Masanao Miyoshi. 2006. "Thermal and Mechanical Properties of Plasticized Poly (L-lactide) Nanocomposites with Organo-modified Montmorillonites." *Journal of Applied Polymer Science* 99 (5). Wiley Online Library: 2594–2602.

Sinclair, R G. 1996. "The Case for Polylactic Acid as a Commodity Packaging Plastic." *Journal of Macromolecular Science, Part A: Pure and Applied Chemistry* 33 (5). Taylor & Francis: 585–97.

Sinha Ray, Suprakas, Pralay Maiti, Masami Okamoto, Kazunobu Yamada, and Kazue Ueda. 2002. "New Polylactide/Layered Silicate Nanocomposites. 1. Preparation, Characterization, and Properties." *Macromolecules* 35 (8). ACS Publications: 3104–10.

Sinha Ray, Suprakas, Kazunobu Yamada, Masami Okamoto, Akinobu Ogami, and Kazue Ueda. 2003. "New Polylactide/Layered Silicate Nanocomposites. 3. High-Performance Biodegradable Materials." *Chemistry of Materials* 15 (7). ACS Publications: 1456–65.

Sinha Ray, Suprakas, Kazunobu Yamada, Masami Okamoto, and Kazue Ueda. 2002. "Polylactide-Layered Silicate Nanocomposite: A Novel Biodegradable Material." *Nano Letters* 2 (10). American Chemical Society: 1093–96. doi:10.1021/nl0202152.

Thellen, Christopher, Caitlin Orroth, Danielle Froio, David Ziegler, Jeanne Lucciarini, Richard Farrell, Nandika Ann D'Souza, and Jo Ann Ratto. 2005. "Influence of Montmorillonite Layered Silicate on Plasticized Poly (l-Lactide) Blown Films." *Polymer* 46 (25). Elsevier: 11716–27.

Tsuji, Hideto, and Yoshito Ikada. 1998. "Blends of Aliphatic Polyesters. II. Hydrolysis of Solution-cast Blends from Poly (L-lactide) and Poly (E-caprolactone) in Phosphate-buffered Solution." *Journal of Applied Polymer Science* 67 (3). Wiley Online Library: 405–15.

Vaia, Richard A, and Emmanuel P Giannelis. 2001. "Polymer Nanocomposites: Status and Opportunities." *MRS Bulletin* 26 (5). Cambridge University Press: 394–401.

Wang, De-Yi, Uwe Gohs, Nian-Jun Kang, Andreas Leuteritz, Regine Boldt, Udo Wagenknecht, and Gert Heinrich. 2012. "Method for Simultaneously Improving the Thermal Stability and Mechanical Properties of Poly(Lactic Acid): Effect of High-Energy Electrons on the Morphological, Mechanical, and Thermal Properties of PLA/MMT Nanocomposites." *Langmuir* 28 (34). American Chemical Society: 12601–8. doi:10.1021/la3025099.

Zheng, Xiaotong, Shaobing Zhou, Yu Xiao, Xiongjun Yu, Xiaohong Li, and Peizhuo Wu. 2009. "Shape Memory Effect of Poly(d,l-Lactide)/Fe3O4 Nanocomposites by Inductive Heating of Magnetite Particles." *Colloids and Surfaces B: Biointerfaces* 71 (1): 67–72. doi: https://doi.org/10.1016/j.colsurfb.2009.01.009.

In: Biocomposites in Bio-Medicine
Editors: Mudasir Ahmad et al.
ISBN: 978-1-53616-247-9
© 2019 Nova Science Publishers, Inc.

Chapter 5

POLYSACCHARIDES BASED NANOCOMPOSITES FOR DRUG DELIVERY SYSTEM

*Anurakshee Verma**
School of Pharmacy, Lingayas University, Faridabad, Haryana, India

ABSTRACT

The design and synthesis of biomaterials with a novel combination is expected to expand the scope of drug-delivery systems in the future. This chapter will focus on the chemical nature of biomaterials as well as the methods used to characterize them with regard to drug delivery. Recent developments in biomaterials capable of intracellular delivery are surveyed to highlight the frontier areas of drug delivery.

Keywords: polysaccharides, drug release system, nanomaterial

---

* Corresponding Author's Email: anurakshee@gmail.com.

1. Introduction of Polysaccharides

Saccharides are generally recognized as carbohydrates. The most simple carbohydrates are *monosaccharide,* which contains a small chain of aldehydes and ketones having hydroxyl groups that have formula $(CH_2O)_n$ where n is three or more monosaccharides are glucose, fructose, and glyceraldehyde (IUPAC 1997). Monosaccharides are the structure blocks of disaccharides that contain a chain of sucrose and lactose. An oligosaccharide is having a small number (3 to 9) sugar or (mono-saccharides). *Oligosaccharides* can have many features, they are normally found on the plasma membrane of animal cells.

Polysaccharides contain more than ten monosaccharide units. Polysaccharides have a general molecular formula of $C_x (H_2O)_y$ where x is usually a large number between 200 and 2500. These repeating units in the polymer backbone are often six-carbon monosaccharides. *Polysaccharides* are having polymeric carbohydrate structure, formed by repeating units of monosaccharides and disaccharides which joined together by glycosidic. They have a structure of monosaccharide from linear to highly branch.

Polysaccharides are an important branch of biological polymers. The function of polysaccharides in living creatures is usually either structure or storage polysaccharides.

- *Storage polysaccharides:* this type of polysaccharide contains starch and glycogen in plants and found in the form of both amylose and the branched amylopectin. In case of animals, found the structurally similar glucose polymer is the more densely branched glycogen, which known as animal starch. Glycogen properties permitted it to be metabolized more quickly, which outfits the active lives of moving animals. Starch and glycogen polysaccharides are called storage polysaccharides because they are stored in the muscles and liver, are converted to energy body functions. Starch is obtained from plants whereas glycogen is obtained from animals.
- *Structural polysaccharides*: this type of polysaccharide contains cellulose and chitin. Cellulose is said to be the most abundant

organic molecule on earth and is used in the cell walls of plants and other organisms (IUPAC 1997). It has wide applications such as paper and textile industries and is also used for the production of rayon, celluloid, cellulose acetate, and nitrocellulose. Chitin has the same structural formula but has nitrogen-containing side branches, that why it increases strength. Chitin found in arthropod exoskeletons and cell walls of fungi. It also has multiple uses, including surgical threads. Callose or laminarin, chrysolaminarin, xylan, arabinoxylan, mannan, fucoidan, and galactomannan are also found in polysaccharides.

Polysaccharides are generally heterogeneous, covering minor modifications of the repeating unit. Depend on the structure; these macromolecules can have different properties from their monosaccharide arrangement. They may be amorphous or even insoluble in water (Metthews 1999). When polysaccharide is having the same type of monosaccharides, this type of polysaccharide is called *homopolysaccharide* or *homoglycan*, but when a different type of monosaccharide is present they are called *heteropolysaccharides* or *heteroglycans* (Campbell 1996; Varki 1999).

Nutrition polysaccharides having common sources of energy. Some micro-organisms can basically degrade starch into glucose but cellulose or other polysaccharides like chitin and arabinoxylans cannot metabolize easily. These polysaccharides can be metabolized by bacteria and protists. These multi-faceted polysaccharides are not digestible, they provide important dietary elements for humans. Depend on these properties it's also called dietary fiber, these carbohydrates type polysaccharides enhance digestion among other benefits (Martin and David 2005). Soluble fiber binds to bile acids in the small intestine, restricted them enter the body, that why turn lowers cholesterol levels in the blood (Weickert and Pfeiffer 2008). After eating, soluble fiber also decreases the absorption of sugar and normalizes blood lipid levels, once fermented in the colon, and produces short-chain fatty acids as byproducts with different physiological activities. Although insoluble fiber is allied with reduced diabetes risk (Scientific Opinion 2010).

Dietary fiber is most important for the diet, with a regulatory establishment in many developed countries (Anderson et al. 2009; Jones and Varady 2015). Dietary fibers are a family of biopolymers, nucleic acids, proteins, and polysaccharides (Weickert and Pfeiffer 2008). Mostly polysaccharides are found easily, expensively recovered natural and produced as energy storage or structural biopolymers by microbes, plants, and animals (Scientific Opinion 2010). Polysaccharides have number of advantages over nucleic acids and proteins for applications in materials science. Polysaccharides are generally more stable than nucleic acids and proteins and are usually not irreversibly denatured on heating (Scientific Opinion 2010).

2. FUNCTIONS OF POLYSACCHARIDES

2.1. Homopolysaccharides

- **Starch:** starch is known as storage polysaccharide and found in plant cells shown in Figure 1. It's having two forms, first is amylose is the helical form of starch comprised only of alpha-1,4 linkages and second is amylopectin that has a structure like glycogen except that the branched alpha-1,6 linkage is present on only about one in 30 monomers.

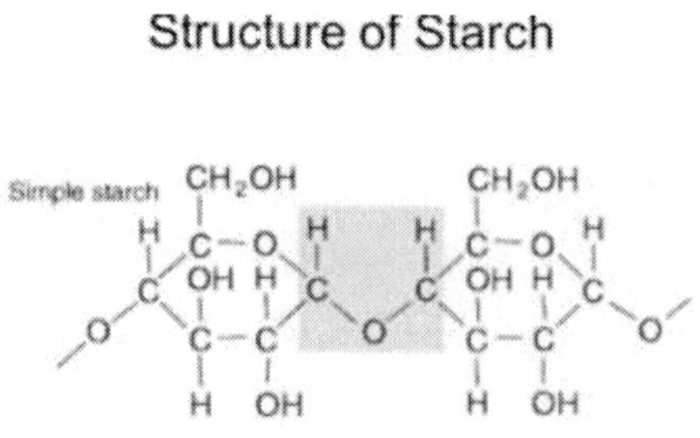

Structure of Starch

Figure 1. Structure of starch.

- **Glycogen:** Glycogen is also known as storage polysaccharides and it's found in animals (Figure 2). It is composed of alpha-1,4-

glycosidic bonds with branched alpha-1,6 bonds present at about every tenth monomer. It is mainly produced by the liver and muscles, but it can also be made during a process called glycogenesis.

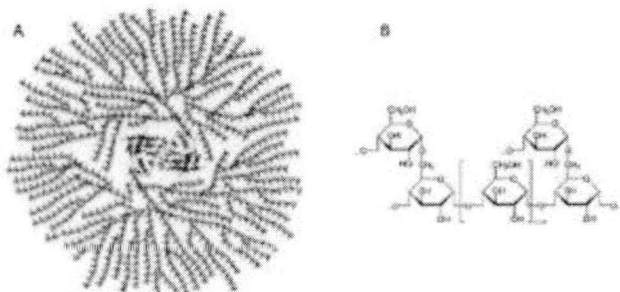

Figure 2. Structure of glycogen.

- **Cellulose:** Cellulose is a structural polysaccharide that is found in the cell wall of plants and when consumed, it acts as a dietary fiber. Cellulose is known as at most plentiful organic molecule on earth. Wood paper and cotton are common forms of cellulose.

2.2. Heteropolysaccharide

Heteropolysaccharides are found in different structural and functional roles in the human body.

- **Dermatan sulfate:** Dermatan sulfate is originated mainly in the skin, and also present in vessels, heart, lungs. It may be related to coagulation and vascular diseases and different conditions.
- **Hyaluronic Acid:** Hyaluronic acid acts as a lubricant and its presence in the synovial fluid of joints.
- **Heparin:** Heparin presents as an anticoagulant in the blood.

- **Chondroitin Sulfate:** Chondroitin sulfate contributes to tensile strength and elasticity of different parts such as walls of the aorta, cartilages, ligament, and tendons.
- **Keratan sulfate:** Keratan sulfate present in the cornea, bone, cartilage and a variety of other body parts such as hair and nails.

In this way, different type of polysaccharides that are present in the human body is glucose-amino-glycans or mucopolysaccharides that are created by the endoplasmic reticulum. Polysaccharides from important material such as connective tissues, collagen, and elastin.

3. Drug Delivery System

The drug delivery system is medium for transporting a pharmaceutical compound (drug) in the particular part of body as desirable to safely release its needed target site with therapeutic effect (Jones and Varady 2015). Drug delivery technologies adapted drug release profile, distribution, absorption, and elimination for the advantage of refining product safety, and efficacy, as well as patient compliance and convenience. Drug release is from diffusion, degradation, swelling, and affinity-based mechanisms. In present time polysaccharides nanoparticle has most attention as a potential drug release system, it's applicable for controlled release of drugs in target site (Aminabhavi et al. 2001). Some of the polysaccharides such as chitosan and deacylated product of chitin have shown best drug release properties. It is insoluble at natural and alkaline pH values but forms salt with inorganic and organic compounds. Upon dissolution the amino groups of chitosan get protonated then polymer became positive charged (Neil 2010). Peptides, antibody, protein, gene and vaccine-based drugs, may not be transported by above routes because due to molecular size and charge issues they cannot be absorbed into the systemic circulation efficiently for therapeutically effective. In this way, many proteins and peptide drugs have to be transported by injection or a nano-carrier technique (Wang and von Recum 2011).

The drug release system can be made by slowly degradable, stimuli reactive (temperature and pH-sensitive) by conjugating them. The targeted drug release system is the ability to direct interest with the drug-loaded system. Two major mechanisms addressing the desired site for drug release (Reddy 2010). Colloidal drug release systems like as micellar solutions, liquid crystal dispersion, Vesicle and nanoparticle dispersion obtain a small particle in the range of 1-400 nm show ideal drug delivery system. This system also modified and achieved goal for drug release systems with optimized drug loading and release properties, long shelf-life and low toxicity (Mueller 2004). Present research in the field of drug delivery includes the development of different types of drug delivery, such as targeted delivery in which the drug is only active in the target area of the body such as in cancerous tissues (Mueller 2004). Sustained drug release, in which the drug is released over a period of time in a controlled way, and methods to enhanced survival of oral agents which must pass through the acidic environment of a stomach (Bertrand and Leroux 2005). Different types of sustained-release formulations were investigated such as include liposomes, drug-loaded biodegradable microspheres, and drug-polymer conjugates and hydrogel (Staff 2015).

4. CLASSIFICATION OF DRUG DELIVERY SYSTEM

Different types of drug delivery systems were investigated, which are following.

- Magnetic drug delivery
- Thin-film drug delivery
- Biodegradable polymer-based drug delivery system
- Bovine submaxillary mucin coatings
- Acoustic targeted drug delivery
- Self-micro emulsifying drug delivery system
- Neural drug delivery systems

5. Polysaccharides Based Drug Delivery System

The field of drug delivery has given a solution to the limited efficacy and high toxicity of many drugs. Nano-sized drug carriers are popular because their size allows for selective accumulation in the diseased area. Polysaccharides are non-toxic and biodegradable natural polymers that can serve as the basis for these nano-sized carriers. Polysaccharide with strong hydrophilicity that may reduce uptake by the reticuloendothelial system and prolong drug circulation.

5.1. Starch-Based Nanoparticle for Drug Delivery System

Starch is a naturally occurring polymeric material, it's extracted from seeds, tubers or roots. Starch shows the chain structure of glucose which linkage by glycoside. It has two forms are amylase which is linear and other is amylopectin's which have branched. In the present time, starch-based hydrogel represents best in drug delivery, tissue engineering, and other biomedical applications (Sa-Lima et al. 2010) developed injectable hydrogels of starch and encapsulated the starch-based gels derived stromal cells for the regeneration of articular cartilage. Chitosan β-glycerophosphate starch hydrogels can be investigated use of chondrogenic and differentiation of ADSC for cartilage regeneration. Hydrogels of starch have found their use in wound dressing (Pal et al. 2006). Investigated transparent starch-based hydrogel membranes, and it's prepared by cross-linking of polyvinyl alcohol with heat-treated corn starch suspension. Nanoparticles intercalated hydrogel matrix shows the unique physicochemical characteristic properties of hydrogels such as thermal, mechanical, barrier, optical, sound, electric simulations, etc. (Schexnailder and Schmidt 009). The aggregation properties are shown by nanoparticles, which are neither stabilized nor charged. Charged nanoparticles may occur exfoliation in water, due to the colloidal interactions of silicates and stabilize the gel formed. Literature review and some new publications covers the synthesis, characterization, and applications of hydrogels of polymer nano-composite covering magnetic and inorganic nanoparticles (Razmjou et al. 2013, Hou et al. 2008, Takahashi et al. 2005) has shown that a modified polyethylene dioxide–laponite system can be investigated for a drug delivery system at physiological situations. A broader variety of applications is mentioned for starch made from nanoparticulate bentonites (natural layered silicate) and PEO polymer. Metal nanoparticles dispersed within hydrogels of polymer nanocomposites can enhance anti-microbial properties and electrical conductance (Murali et al. 2007, Kozlovskaya et al. 2008). Gaharwar (2011) were investigated Polymer–magnetic nanocomposites, with particles in the polymer matrix dispersed within cross-linking polymer chains (Gaharwar et al. 2001). PEG and silicate nanoparticles synthesized nanocomposite hydrogel. Recent research demonstrated the potential of silicate-PEG nanocomposite hydrogels in craniofacial, orthopedic and dental applications. Viscosity measurements for the function of shear rates represented in Figure 3.

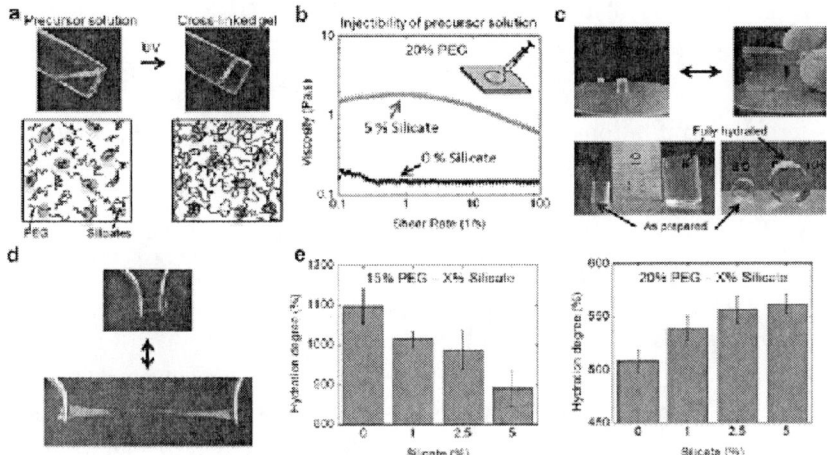

Figure 3. Transparent PEG–silicate nanocomposite hydrogels.

Synthesized nanocomposite observed the result that nanocomposites were used for sustaining the extreme mechanical deformation. The swelling characteristics of the nanocomposites were affected by the ratio of silicate nanocomposites. Many other aspects of polymer nanocomposites are currently being investigated, such as the effects of nano-filler on chain dynamics, and it depends on the final properties and degree of dispersion. Ideal hydrogels have been synthesized by direct dissolution of chitin at low temperatures. A clear transparent solution in a mixture of 8wt%NaOH/4wt% urea aqueous solution by freeze/thawing method to prepare transparently (Chang et al. 2011). The chitin hydrogels may find wide use in bio-applications, as a result of the more stable structure and better compatibility of chitin than its derivatives (Chang et al. 2011). Hydrogel nanocomposites are also being investigated as pressure-sensitive adhesives for skin contact applications. Monodisperse polystyrene nanoparticle used as a filler on the network formation, rheological properties and adhesion performance of hydrogel nanocomposites (Bait et al. 2011). Organically modified phyllosilicate form organoclay, which derived from the naturally occurring clay mineral. Polydimethylsiloxane (PDMS) intercalated organoclay shows the results in the formation of pressure-sensitive adhesives. Shaikh (2007) obtained the partially exfoliated nanocomposites of PDMS. It was shown that different ratios of the organo-silicate additive to the polymer matrix, nanocomposites enhanced the drug release kinetics and the adhesive properties of the matrix (Shaikh et al. 2007). Present emphasis is to develop transdermal formulations, which are based on natural polymer matrix and for better release technologies in, which the dispersion of the drug is uniform within the transdermal layer (Brown et al. 2006; Naik et al. 2000).

5.2. Cellulose Based Drug Delivery System

Cellulose is mostly known as naturally occurring polysaccharides and its derivatives have been broadly used in the pharmaceutical field as drug delivery. Hydroxyl propyl cellulose was synthesized and modifying by some of the cellulose hydroxyl groups with propylene oxide to enhance the cellulose solubility and control drug release (Kamel et al. 2008). Which improves the oral delivery of hydrophobic drugs, which often have less bioavailability after administration, Winnik (2003) Modified hydroxyl propyl cellulose with hydrophobic hexadecyl or octadecyl groups through polyoxyethylene linker of variable length (Francis et al. 2003). Five hydrophobic molecules were attached to one hydroxyl propyl cellulose chain, the critical micelle concentration was 65–135 mg/L while with ten hydrophobic chains, the critical micelle concentration dropped to 15–22 mg/L. Less water-soluble immunosuppressant (Cyclosporin A), was used as ideal drug. The maximum loading was 0.025 mg CyA/mg micelle was observed with lower hydrophobic modification, while, as anticipated, with higher modification and loading capacity increased to 0.067 mg CyA/mg micelle. PEO-C16 provided an improved solubilizing environment for CyA relative to PEO-C18 with the same quantity of hydrophobic moieties. The polymeric micelles size dropped from 78–90 nm to 44–74 nm by the encapsulation of CyA. Presumably, the encapsulation of CyA enhances the hydrophobic interactions in the core and produces more compact particles. In vitro-studies showed HPC-PEO-C16 micellar system had high affinity to mucus and could enhance the permeability of entrapped therapeutics across intestine epithelial-Caco-2 cells (Xiong et al. 2012; Chayed et al. 2003; Francis et al. 2005; Enomoto-Rogers et al.2011; Clagett et al. 1998; Francis et al. 2003; Francis et al. 2005; Yuan et al. 2006; Xu et al. 2006; Houga et al. 2009; Daoud-Mahammed et al. 2009). These studies demonstrated the great potential of cellulose-based micelles for improved oral delivery of hydrophobic drugs. A literature review has focused on the design and synthesis of cellulose-based micelles; such systems include HPC-polycaprolactone (Discher and Ahmed. 2006) and cellulose-C15-pyrene micelle. Micelles prepared from cellulose-C15-pyrene with longer cellulose chains and smaller in size relative to those prepared from short-chain cellulose and shows multilayer micelle (Chen et al. 2006). *Galkina* et al. synthesized TiO2 modified nanocomposite based on cellulose nanofibers and loaded three types of medicines, diclofenac sodium, penicillamine-D, and phosphomycin. Diclofenac released was observed fast and highest about 90% within 70 minutes (Enomoto-Rogers et al. 2011).

Many researchers are also developing as promising polysaccharides carriers for drug delivery systems with the present improvement and breakthrough of the nanocellulose modification techniques, at present time nano cellulose are drawing wonderful attentions in drug delivery systems and continue to grow positive result (Galkina et al. 2015; Peng et al. 2011; Habibi et al. 2010). Das (2012) synthesized cellulose nano-whiskers for a novel drug delivery system (Das et al. 2012). That was adapted for the controlled delivery of enzymes, proteins and amine-containing drugs with the selection of desired linker molecules. Representing the processes exist between sources of bacterial cellulose and its drug delivery system in Figure 4.

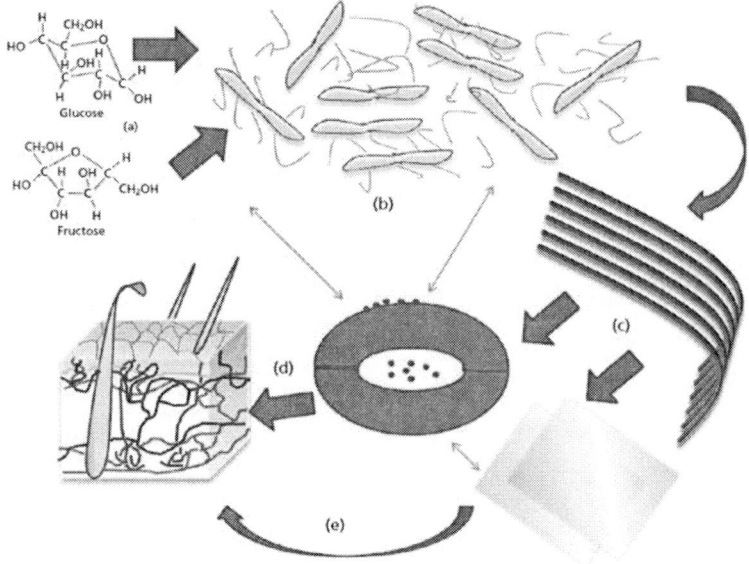

Figure 4. Representation of processes ranging between sources of bacterial cellulose and its drug delivery system.

5.3. Chitosan Based Drug Delivery System

In current times chitosan and its derivatives have been most broadly investigated composites for drug delivery due to valuable properties. Many researchers have focused on chitosan-based drug delivery systems (Figure 5) for improvement of hydrophobic drug delivery. Most of these systems were developed by chitosan and its derivative with hydrophobic moieties such as stearic acid (Xie et al. 2006; Du et al. 2011; Hu et al. 2009; Hu et

2008; Hu et al. 2012), deoxycholic acid (Hu et al. 2012; Jin et al. 2012; Lee et al. 2012; Wang et al.2012), glycyrrhetinic acid (Tian et al. 2012), polycaprolactone (Zhang et al. 2011; Chen et al. 2011). Modified chitosan can lead to the formation of self-assemble spherical nano and macro composites with a range of 20–500 nm in aqueous solution. Modification percentage of higher hydrophobic moieties usually gives rise to a smaller composite diameter due to stronger hydrophobic interactions. Several anti-tumor therapeutics such as paclitaxel (Sahu et al. 2011; Mo et al. 2011; Lian et al. 2011), doxorubicin (Huo et al. 2012; Jin et al. 2012; Du et al. 2011; Du et al. 2011; Srinophakun and Boonmee. 2012; Du et al. 2012), and camptothec in Du (2012), have been used as ideal drugs which encapsulated by chitosan modified composite. The chitosan modified nano and micro composite enhanced the solubility of the hydrophobic drugs and these composites showed controlled or sustained release of the hydrophobic drugs. A higher degree of substitution usually specified slower drug release despite insignificant changes in the loading efficiency. The therapeutic-loaded nano and micro composites showed significantly higher toxicity to tumor cells for in vitro compared to free drugs due to improved drug internalization. Chitosan-based composites have been used to improve oral drug delivery due to muco and bioadhesive nature of chitosan. Chitosan-based composites were established to inhibit the activity of P-glycoprotein 1 ATPase (Jiang et al.2011). Chitosan has opened the tight junctions between cells, in this reason it has greater drug absorption capacity. The chitosan-based composites were characterized by low CMCs, for high stability (Sonaje et al.2011) and resistance to the harsh environment of the gastrointestinal tract. N-octyl-O-sulfate chitosan can improve the oral bioavailability of PTX (Srinophakun and Boonmee .2012).

Chitosan-based materials were established to be a relatively safe vehicle of a drug for oral formulation (Lin et al. 2011). Chitosan-based drug release systems have also been examined for applications in antivirus (Sonaje et al. 2011), anti-thrombogenicity (Lin et al. 2011), and anti-platelet aggregation release (Jiang et al. 2011).

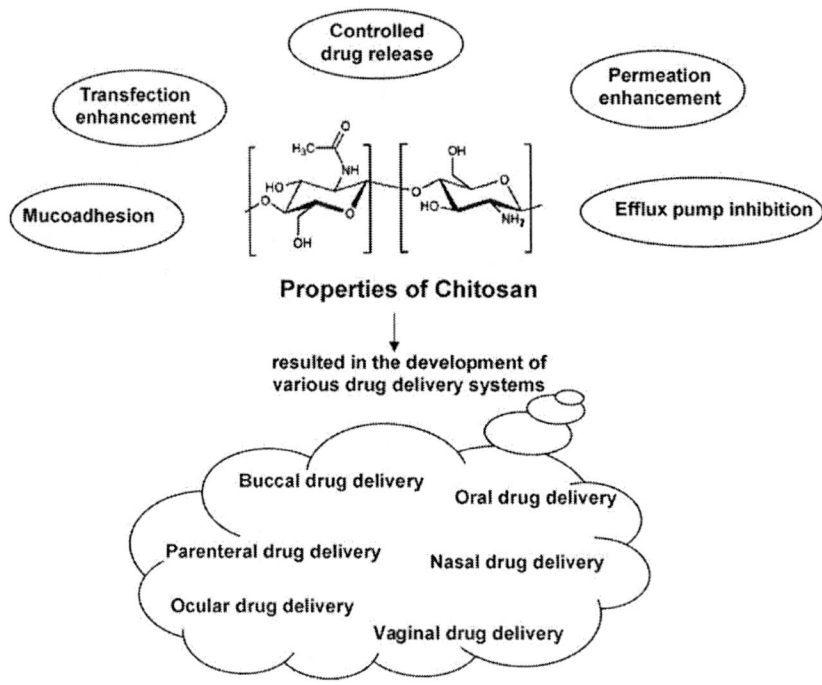

Figure 5. Chitosan-based drug delivery systems.

CONCLUSION

Polysaccharides based drug delivery systems have shown potential improvement of drug and protein delivery by enhanced solubility, stability, and controllable drug release properties. Polysaccharide-based drug release system was also shown prolonged circulation and favorable pharmacokinetics in several models, indicating the potential for translation to clinical research. Polysaccharide-based drug delivery system forms a clear trend towards more complex and controllable systems, which will possess higher targeting and specificity to further improve therapeutic efficacy and reduce undesired side effects. Polysaccharide possesses some very extraordinary properties which make it a very useful biomaterial for drug delivery includes its biocompatibility, absorbability on biological membranes, no antigenicity, low toxicity, synergism with other bioactive compounds, etc. This advantage will value the future development of biomaterial for drug delivery.

REFERENCES

Bait Nadia, Bruno Grassl, Christophe Derail, Ahmad Benaboura. 2011 "Hydrogel nanocomposites as pressure-sensitive adhesives for skin-contact applications" *Soft Matterial* 7: 2025-2032.

Bertrand Nicolas, Jean-Christophe Leroux. 2015 "The journey of a drug carrier in the body: an anatomo-physiological perspective" *Journal of Controlled Release* 161: 152–63.

Brown, Marc B, Martin, Gary P., Jones, Stuart A., Akomeah, Franklin K. 2006 "Dermal and transdermal drug delivery systems: Current and future prospects" *Drug delivery* 13:175-187.

Chang, Chunyu, Chen, Si, Zhang, Lina. 2011 "Novel hydrogels prepared via direct dissolution of chitin at low temperature: structure and biocompatibility" *Journal of Materials Chemistry* 21:3865-3871.

Chawan, Manaspon, Viravaidya-Pasuwat, Kwanchanok, Pimpha, Nuttaporn. 2012 "Preparation of folate-conjugated pluronic f127/chitosan core-shell nanoparticles encapsulating doxorubicin for breast cancer treatment" *Journal of Nanomaterials* 2012, 2012, 593878:1–593878:11.

Chayed, S., Winnik, F. M. 2007 "In vitro evaluation of the mucoadhesive properties of polysaccharide-based nanoparticulate oral drug delivery systems" *European Journal of Pharmaceutics and Biopharmaceutics* 65:363–370.

Chen, C. H., Cuong, N. V., Chen, Y. T., So, R. C., Liau, I., Hsieh, M. F. 2011 "Overcoming multidrug resistance of breast cancer cells by the micellar doxorubicin nanoparticles of mPEG-PCL-graft-cellulose" *Jouranal of Nanoscience Nanotechnology* 11:53–60.

Chen, C., Cai, G. Q., Zhang, H. W., Jiang, H. L., Wang, L. Q. 2011 "Chitosan-poly(epsiloncaprolactone)- poly(ethylene glycol) graft copolymers: Synthesis, self-assembly, and drug release behavior" *Journal of Biomedical Materials Research Part A*. 96A:116–124.

Clagett, G. P., Anderson, F. A., Geerts, W, Heit, J. A., Knudson, M., Lieberman, J. R., Merli, G. J., Wheele, H. B. 1998 "Prevention of venous thromboembolism" *Chest* 114:531S–560S.

Daoud-Mahammed, S., Couvreur, P., Bouchemal, K., Cheron, M., Lebas, G., Amiel, C, Gref, R. 2009 "Cyclodextrin and polysaccharide-based nanogels: Entrapment of two hydrophobic molecules" benzophenone and tamoxifen. *Biomacromolecules*. 10:547–554.

Dash, Rajalaxmi, Ragauskas, Arthur J. 2012 "Synthesis of a novel cellulose nanowhisker-based drug delivery system" *RSC Advances*, 2:3403-3409.

Discher, D. E., Ahmed, F. 2006 Polymersomes. *Annual Review on Biomedical Engineering* 8:323–341.

Du YZ, L Wang, H Yuan, FQ Hu. 2011 "Linoleic acid-grafted chitosan oligosaccharide micelles for intracellular drug delivery and reverse drug resistance of tumor cells" *International Journal of Biological Macromolecules* 2011, 48: 215–222.

Du, Y. Z., Cai, L. L., Liu, P., You, J., Yua, H., Hu, F. Q. 2012 "Tumor cells-specific targeting delivery achieved by A54 peptide functionalized polymeric micelles" *Biomaterials*. 33:8858–8867.

Eastwood, Martin, David, Kritchevsky. 2005 "Dietary fiber: how did we get where we are" *Annual Review of Nutrition* 25:1–8.

Enomoto-Rogers, Yukiko, Kamitakahara, Hiroshi, Yoshinaga, Arata, Takano, Toshiyuki. 2011 "Synthesis of diblock copolymers with cellulose derivatives 4. Self-assembled nanoparticles of amphiphilic cellulose derivatives carrying a single pyrene group at the reducing-end" *Cellulose* 18:1005–1014.

Enomoto-Rogers, Yukiko, Kamitakahara, Hiroshi, Yoshinaga, Arata, Takano, Toshiyuki. 2011 "Synthesis of diblock copolymers with cellulose derivatives 4. Self-assembled nanoparticles of amphiphilic cellulose derivatives carrying a single pyrene group at the reducing-end" *Cellulose* 18:1005–1014.

Francis M. F., Cristea, M., Winnik, F. M.. 2005 "Exploiting the vitamin B-12 pathway to enhance oral drug delivery via polymeric micelles" *Biomacromolecules.* 6:2462–2467.

Francis, M. F., Lavoie, L., Winnik, F. M., Leroux, J. C. 2003 "Solubilization of cyclosporin A in dextran-g-polyethyleneglycolalkyl ether polymeric micelle" *European Journal of Pharmaceutics and Biopharmaceutics* 56:337–346.

Francis, M. F., Piredda, M., Winnik, F. M.. 2003 "Solubilization of poorly water soluble drugs in micelles of hydrophobically modified hydroxypropylcellulose copolymers" *Journal Control Release* 93:59–68.

Francis, Mira F., Mariella, Cristea, Yang, Y. L., Winnik, F. M. 2005 "Engineering polysaccharide-based polymeric micelles to enhance permeability of cyclosporin a across Caco-2 cells" *Pharmaceutical Research* 22:209–219.

Gaharwar, Akhilesh K, Rivera, Christian P., Wu, Chia-Jung, Schmidt, Gudrun. 2011 "Transparent, elastomeric and tough hydrogels from poly(ethylene glycol) and silicate nanoparticles" *Acta Biomaterialia* 7:4139-4148.

Galkina, O. L., Ivanov V. K., Agafonov A. V., Seisenbaeva, G. A., Kessler V. G. J. 2015 "Cellulose nanofiber–titania nanocomposites as potential drug delivery systems for dermal applications" *Journal of Material Chemistry B* 3:1688-1698.

Habibi Youssef, Lucian A Lucia, Ornaldo J Rojas. 2010 "Cellulose Nanocrystals: Chemistry, Self-Assembly, and Applications" *Chemical Review* 110:3479–3500.

Helena, Sá-Lima, Caridade, Sofia G., Mano, João F., Reis, Rui L. 2010 "Stimuli-responsive chitosan-starch injectable hydrogels combined with encapsulated adipose-derived stromal cells for articular cartilage regeneration" *Soft Matterial* 6:5184-5195.

Houga, C., J. Giermanska, S. Lecommandoux, R. Borsali, D. Taton, Y. Gnanou, J. F. Le Meins. 2009 "Micelles and polymersomes obtained by self-assembly of dextran and polystyrene based blockcopolymers" *Biomacromolecules.*10:32–40.

Hu Fu-Qiang, Chen, W. W., Zhao, M. D., Yuan, H., Du, Y. Z. 2012 "Effective antitumor gene therapy delivered by polyethylenimine-conjugated stearic acid-g-chitosan oligosaccharide micelles" *Gene Therapy* 20: 597-606

Hu Fu-Qiang, Jiang, X. H, Huang, X., Wu, X. L., Hong Yuan, Wei, X. H, Yong-Zhong Du. 2009 "Enhanced cellular uptake of chlorine e6 mediated by stearic acid-grafted chitosan oligosaccharide micelles" *Journal of Drug Target* 17:384–391.

Hu Fu-Qiang, Wu, X. L., Du, Yong-Zhong, You, J., Yuan, Hong. 2008 "Cellular uptake and cytotoxicity of shell crosslinked stearic acid-grafted chitosan oligosaccharide micelles encapsulating doxorubicin" *European Journal of Pharmaceutics and Biopharmaceutics* 69:117–125.

Huo M., Zou, A. Yao, C., Zhang, Y, Zhou, J., Wang, J., Zhu, Q., Li, J., Q Zhang. 2012 "Somatostatin receptor-mediated tumor-targeting drug delivery using octreotide-PEG-deoxycholic acid conjugate-modified N-deoxycholic acid-O,N-hydroxyethylation chitosan micelles" *Bio materials* 2012, 33: 6393–6407.

IUPAC, 1997. Compendium of Chemical Terminology (Gold Book, 2nd ed.) Online corrected version: (2006)" heteropolysaccharide (heteroglycan).

IUPAC. 1997. Compendium of Chemical Terminology (Gold Book, 2nd ed.) Online corrected version: (2006) homopolysaccharide (homoglycan).

James W. Anderson, Pats Baird, Richard, H. Davis. 2009 "Health benefits of dietary fiber" *Nutrition Review* 67:188–205.

Jiang G. B., Lin, Z. T., Xu, X. J. Zhang, H., Song, K. 2012 "Stable nanomicelles based on chitosan derivative: In vitro antiplatelet aggregation and adhesion properties" *Carbohydrate Polymer*, 88:232–238.

Jin, Y. H., Hu H. Y., Qiao, M. X., Zhu, J., Qi, J. W., Hu, C. J., Zhang, Q, Chen, D, W. 2012 "pH-Sensitive chitosan-derived nanoparticles as doxorubicin carriers for effective anti-tumor activity: Preparation and in vitro evaluation" *Colloids Surfaces B Biointerfaces* 94:184–191.

Jin, Y. H., Hu, H. Y., Qiao, M. X., Zhu, J., Qi, J. W., Hu, C. J., Zhang Q., Chen, D. W. 2012 "pH-Sensitive chitosan-derived nanoparticles as doxorubicin carriers for effective anti-tumor activity: Preparation and in vitro evaluation" *Colloids Surfaces B Biointerfaces* 94:184–191.

Jones Peter, J, Varady, Krista A.. 2015 "Are functional foods redefining nutritional requirements". *Applied Physiology Nutrition and Metabolism* 33:118–23.

Kamel, S., Ali, N., Jahangir, K., Shah, S. M., El-Gendy, A. A. 2008 "Pharmaceutical significance ofcellulose: A review" *Express Polymer Letter*2:758–778.

Kozlovskaya Veronika, Kharlampieva, Eugenia, Khanal, Bishnu P., Pramit Manna, Zubarev, Eugene R., Tsukruk, Vladimir V. 2008 "Ultrathin Layer-by-Layer Hydrogels with Incorporated Gold Nanorods as pH-Sensitive Optical Materials" *Chemistry of materials* 20:7474-7485.

Kunal, Pal, Banthia, Ajit, Majumdar, Deepak K.. 2006 "Preparation of transparent starch based hydrogel membrane with potential application as wound dressing" *Trends Biomaterial Artificial Organs* 20:59-67.

Lee, J, Lee, C, Kim T. H., Lee E. S., Shin B. S., Chi, S. C., Park, E. S., Lee, K. C., Youn Y. S.. 2012 "Self-assembled glycol chitosan nanogels containing palmityl-acylated exendin-4 peptide as a long-acting anti-diabetic inhalation system" *Journal of Control Release* 161:728–734.

Li Z. G., Li, X. Y., Cao ZX, Xu, YZ, Lin HJ, Zhao YL, Wei Y. Q., Qian Z. Y. 2012 "Camptothecin nanocolloids based on N,N,N-trimethyl chitosan: Efficient suppression of growth of multiple myeloma in a murine model" *Oncology Report*, 27:1035–1040.

Lian, H., Sun, J., Yu, Y. P., Liu, YH, Cao, W., Wang, Y. J., Sun, Y. H., Wang, S. L., He, Z. G. 2011 "Supramolecular micellar nanoaggregates based on a novel chitosan/vitamin E succinate copolymer for paclitaxel selective delivery" *International Journal of Nanomedicine* 6: 3323–3334.

Lin, Z. T., Song, K., Bin, J. P., Liao, Y. L., Jiang, G. B.. 2011 "Characterization of polymer micelles with hemocompatibility based on N-succinyl-chitosan grafting with long chain hydrophobic groups and loading aspirin" *Journal of Material Chemistry.* 21:19153–19165.

Matthews, C. E., Holde, K. E. Van, Ahern, K. G. 1999. Biochemistry (3rd edition) New York: Benjamin Cummings.

Mo R., Jin X., N. L., Ju, C. Y., Sun, M. J., Zhang. C, Ping, Q. N. 2011 "The mechanism of enhancement on oral absorption of paclitaxel by N-octyl-O-sulfate chitosan micelles" *Biomaterial* 32:4609–4620.

Mueller-Goymann, Christel. 2004 "Physicochemical characterization of colloidal drug delivery systems such as reverse micelles, vesicles, liquid crystals and nanoparticles for topical administration," European *Journal of Pharmaceutics and Biopharmaceutics* 58,2: 343-356.

Murali Mohan Y, Lee, K, Premkumar T., Geckeler, K. E., 2007 "Hydrogel networks as nanoreactors: a novel approach to silver nanoparticles for antibacterial applications" *Polymer* 48:158-164.

N. A., Campbell. 1996. Biology (4th edition) New York: Benjamin Cummings.

Naik, A., Kalia Y. N., Guy, R. H. 2000 "Transdermal drug delivery: overcoming the skin's barrier function" *Pharmaceutical science & technology today* 3:318-326.

Neil Jacklyn. 2010 "Controlling drug delivery for the application of extended or sustained-release drug products for parenteral administration." *Chemistry Master's Theses., Northeastern University*:14.

Peng, B. L., Dhar, N., Liu, H. L., Tam, K. C. 2011 "Chemistry and applications of nanocrystalline cellulose and its derivatives: A nanotechnology perspective" *Canadian Journal of Chemical Engineering* 9999:1–16.

Razmjou Amir, Mohammad Reza Barati, George P Simon, Kiyonori Suzuki, Huanting Wang. 2013 "Fast Deswelling of Nanocomposite Polymer Hydrogels via Magnetic Field-Induced Heating for Emerging FO Desalination" *Environmental science & technology* 12:6297-6305.

Reddy. P. Dwarakanadha, D Swarnalatha 2010 "Recent advances in Novel Drug Delivery Systems" *International Journal of PharmTechResearch* 2: 2025-2027.

Sahu S. K., Maiti, S., Maiti, T. K., Ghosh, S. K., P Pramanik. 2011 "Hydrophobically modified carboxymethyl chitosan nanoparticles targeted delivery of paclitaxel" *Journal of Drug Target* 19:104–113.

Schexnailder, Patrick J., Gudrun Schmidt. 2009 "Nanocomposite polymer hydrogels" *Colloid and Polymer Science* 287:1-11.

Scientific Opinion. 2010. "Scientific Opinion on Dietary Reference Values for carbohydrates and dietary fibre" *European Food Safety Authority Journal* 8: 1462.

Shaikh, Sohel, Anil Birdi, Syed Qutubuddin, Eric Lakatosh, Harihara Baskaran. 2007 Controlled release in transdermal pressure sensitive adhesives using organosilicate nanocomposites. *Annals of biomedical engineering* 35:2130-2137.

Sonaje K., K. J. Lin, MT Tseng, S. P. Wey, F. Y. Su, Chuang, E. Y., Hsu C. W., Chen C. T., Sung, H. W. 2011 "Effects of chitosan-nanoparticle-mediated tight junction opening on the oral absorption of endotoxins" *Biomaterials,* 32:8712–8721.

Soppimath, Kumaresh S, Aminabhavi Tejraj M., Kulkarni Anandrao R., Rudzinski, Walter E. 2001 "Biodegradable polymeric nanoparticles as drug delivery devices" *Journal of Controlled Release* 70:1-20.

Srinophakun Thongchai, Jirapat Boonmee, J. 2011 "Preliminary study of conformation and drug release mechanism of doxorubicin-conjugated glycol chitosan, via cis-aconityl linkage, by molecular modeling" *International Journal Molecular Science* 12:1672–1683.

Staff. 2015. "Acid-friendly Microbe Finds Application in Drug Delivery" *American Laboratory paper* 47: 7

Takahashi Tadahito, Yamada, Yoshiaki, Kataoka, Kazunori, Nagasaki, Yukio. 2005 "Preparation of a novel PEG–clay hybrid as a DDS material: Dispersion stability and sustained release profiles" *Journal of Controlled Release* 107:408-416.

Tian, Q., Wang, X. H., Wang, W., Zhang, C. N., Wang, P., Yuan, Z. 2012 "Self-assembly and liver targeting of sulfated chitosan nanoparticles functionalized with glycyrrhetinic acid" *Nanomedicine Nano technology Biology Medicine* 8:870–879.

Varki, A., Cummings R., Esko, J., Freeze, H., Stanley, P., Bertozzi, C., Hart, G., Etzler, M. 1999 *Essentials of glycobiology*. (2nd edition) Cold Spring Harbor Laboratory New York.

Wang F., Chen, Y., Zhang, D., Zhang, Q., Zheng, D., Hao, L., Liu, Y., Duan, C., Jia, L., Liu, G. 2012 "Folate-mediated targeted and intracellular delivery of paclitaxel using a novel deoxycholic acid-O-carboxymethylated chitosan-folic acid micelles" *International Journal of Nanomedicine* 7:325–337.

Wang X. H., Tian, Q., Wang, W., Zhang, C. N., Wang, P., Yuan, Z. 2012 "In vitro evaluation of polymeric micelles based on hydrophobically-modified sulfated chitosan as a carrier of doxorubicin" *The Journal of Materials Science: Materials in Medicine*. 23:1663–1674.

Wang, Nick X., Recum, Horst A von. 2011 "Affinity-Based Drug Delivery" *Macromolecular Bioscience* 11: 321–332.

Weickert, M. O., Pfeiffer A. F. 2008 "Metabolic effects of dietary fiberand any other substance that consume and prevention of diabetes" *Journal of Nutrition* 138: 439–442.

Xie, Y. T., Du, Yong-Zhong, Yuan, Hong, Hu, Fu-Qiang. 2012 "Brain-targeting study of stearic acid-grafted chitosan micelle drug-delivery system" *International Journal of Nanomedicine* 7:3235–3244.

Xiong, Yubing, Qi, Jianing, Yao, Ping. 2012 "P. Amphiphilic cholic-acid-modified dextran sulfate and its application for the controlled delivery of superoxide dismutase" *Macromolecular Bioscience* 12:515–524.

Xu Qingguo, Xubo Yuan, Jin Chang. 2005 "Self-aggregates of cholic acid hydrazide-dextran conjugates as drug carriers" *Journal of Applied Polymer Science* 95:487–493.

Yaping, Hou, Matthews, Andrew R.. Smitherman, Ashley M., Bulick, Allen S., Hahn, Mariah S., Hou, Huijie, Han, Arum. 2008 "Thermoresponsive nanocomposite hydrogels with cell-releasing behavior" *Biomaterials* 29:3175-3184.

Yong-Zhong, Du, Cai, Li-Li, Li, Jin, Zhao, Meng-Dan, Chen, Feng-Ying, Yuan, Hong, Hu, Fu-Qiang. 2011 "Receptor-mediated gene delivery by folic acid-modified stearic acid-grafted chitosan micelles" *International Journal of Nanomedicine* 6:1559–1568.

Yuan Xu-Bo, Li, Hong, Zhu, Xiao-Xia, Woo, Hee-Gweon. 2006 "Self-aggregated nanoparticles composed of periodate-oxidized dextran and cholic acid: Preparation, stabilization and in-vitro drug release" *Journal of Chemical Technology and Biotechnology* 81:746–754.

Zhang H. W., Cai, G. Q. Tang, G. P., Wang, L. Q., Jiang, H. L. 2011 "Synthesis, self-assembly, and cytotoxicity of well-defined trimethylated chitosan-O-poly(epsilon-caprolactone): Effect of chitosan molecular weight" *Journal of Biomedical Materials Research Part B* 98B, 290–299.

In: Biocomposites in Bio-Medicine
Editors: Mudasir Ahmad et al.
ISBN: 978-1-53616-247-9
© 2019 Nova Science Publishers, Inc.

Chapter 6

POLYVINYL ALCOHOL (PVA) BASED NANOCOMPOSITES FOR BIOMEDICAL AND TISSUE ENGINEERING APPLICATIONS

Sapana Jadoun[1,*] *and Nirmala Kumari Jangid*[2]

[1]School of Basic & Applied Sciences, Department of Chemistry, Lingayas Vidyapeeth, Faridabad, Haryana, India
[2]Department of Chemistry, Banasthali Vidyapith, Rajasthan, India

ABSTRACT

PVA is a synthetic polymer that has been widely used for the last 30 years in the medical, clinically, non-clinically and other fields. In the field of nanocomposites, current research and development are much focused on polymer matrix-based nanocomposites. The aim of the chapter is to explore the synthesis, properties and biomedical applications of polyvinyl alcohol (PVA) based nanocomposites. Such nanocomposites have outstanding thermal stability, mechanical properties, noncarcinogenicity, non-toxicity, biocompatibility, and flexibility. These properties of PVA based nanocomposites makes them a suitable candidate for medicinal and biomedical applications such as drug delivery, wound dressings, soft

---

*Corresponding Author's Email: sjadoun022@ gmail.com.

biomaterial implants and bone tissue engineering. Special focus is given to the biomedical applications of PVA based nanocomposites.

Keywords: polyvinyl alcohol, properties, biocompatibility, biomedical application

INTRODUCTION

Polyvinyl alcohol (PVA) is a synthetic polymer that has been essentially derived from the saponification process of polyvinyl acetate through hydrolysis (Pal, Banthia, and Majumdar 2007; Hill and Le 2001), has been used throughout the first half of the 20th century worldwide. In water, it is a solubilized crystalline structure polymer that is easily degradable by biological organisms having a wide range of applications in commercial, industrial, medical and food areas. Along with these applications, it has been also used in producing end products like food packaging materials, resins, lacquers, surgical threads, etc. PVA is also used as a blending with other polymers having hydrophilic properties (Lee et al., 2004; C. Zhang et al., 2005; Mansur, Oréfice, and Mansur 2004; Xu et al., 2009; Salavagione, Gomez, and Martinez 2009; Hyon, Cha, and Ikada 1989; Mansur et al., 2008; BUNN 1948). It has been also used in many industrial applications for enhancing mechanical strength due to its compatible and hydrophilic nature (Limpan et al., 2012; M. Liu et al., 2007; DeMerlis and Schoneker 2003; Razzak and Darwis 2001) along with its use in nanofillers and crosslinked product (Qiu and Netravali 2013, 2012).

Polymer nanocomposites, ceramic nanocomposites, and metal nanocomposites are the main groups of nanocomposites. Current studies revealed that polymer nanocomposites can be used in several medical areas along with aerospace, packaging, construction, optoelectronic devices, etc. Nanomedicine is the field of diagnosing, curing, treating, preventing diseases as well as dealing with an excruciating injury, alleviating pain and protecting human health with the help of molecular tools and health of the human body (Feldman 2016; Tiwari et al., 2012). A wide variety of nanocomposites based on PVA have been prepared by taking it as a matrix or nano reinforcement like layered silicate. The method of synthesis of these nanocomposites is generally in situ polymerization or solution casting. The first nanocomposite of PVA with a complete range of MMT loading was PVA/MMT nanocomposites. PVA nanocomposites, alpha-chitin whisker reinforced, were prepared with or without heat treatment (X. Zhang et al., 2003; Liang et al., 2009; Roohani et al., 2008; Strawhecker and Manias 2000).

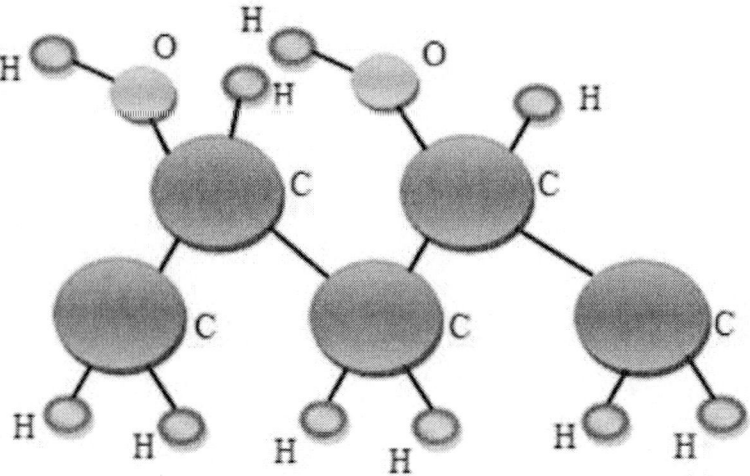

Figure 1. Structure of polyvinyl alcohol (PVA).

METHODS

1. Synthesis of PVA Based Nanocomposites

Ferrite-polymer nanocomposite based on PVA was synthesized by Sindhu (2006) by direct mixing of the PVA and ferrite, followed by sonication. Polyvinyl alcohol (PVA) nanocomposite hydrogels were synthesized by different loading of hydrophilic natural Na-montmorillonite nano clay. Dehydration tests of these nanocomposites were performed and found the direct dependency of these on the dehydration temperature (M

Sirousazar et al., 2011). Nanocomposites of polyvinyl alcohol (PVA) with starch-containing some montmorillonite were prepared by (Spiridon et al., 2008). The enzymatic degradation studies of the above nanocomposites were performed on the basis of determinations of mass loss and the reducing sugars.

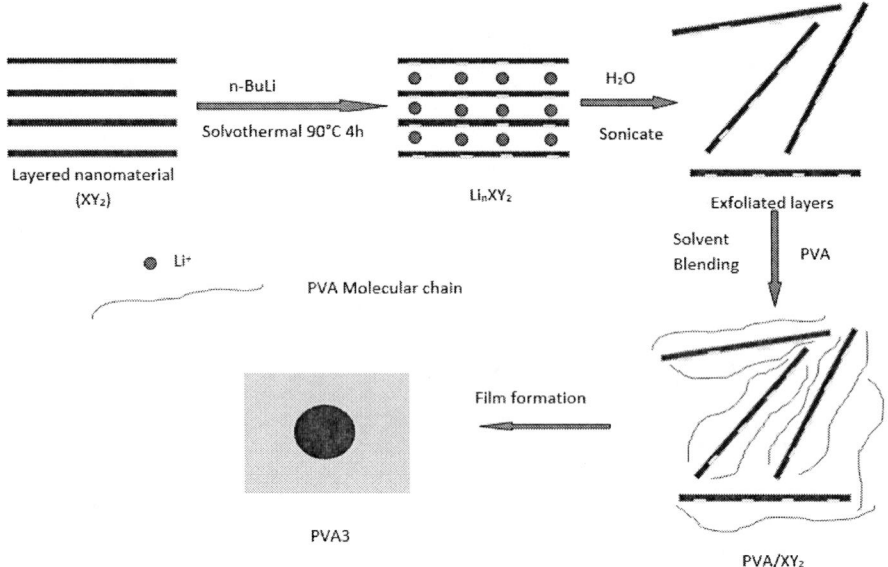

Figure 2. General preparation process of PVA nanocomposites.

2. Properties of PVA Nanocomposites

Recently, K. Zhou (2012) reported that the addition of 1−5 wt. % exfoliated molybdenum disulfide nanosheets in polyvinyl alcohol (PVA), resulted in a nanocomposite with ≈28% enhanced storage modulus with ≈24% increment in the tensile strength. Molybdenum disulfide (MoS_2)/polyvinyl alcohol (PVA) nanocomposites are prepared by Zhou and coworkers (K. Zhou et al., 2012a) via solvent blending method and found the enhancement in the mechanical properties, fire resistance properties and thermal properties which revealed the good dispersion of MoS_2 in PVA and strong interactions between them. Nanocomposites obtained from polyvinyl alcohol (PVA) and cellulose whiskers (CWs) revealed outstanding improvement in mechanical properties (Jalal Uddin, Araki, and Gotoh 2011)

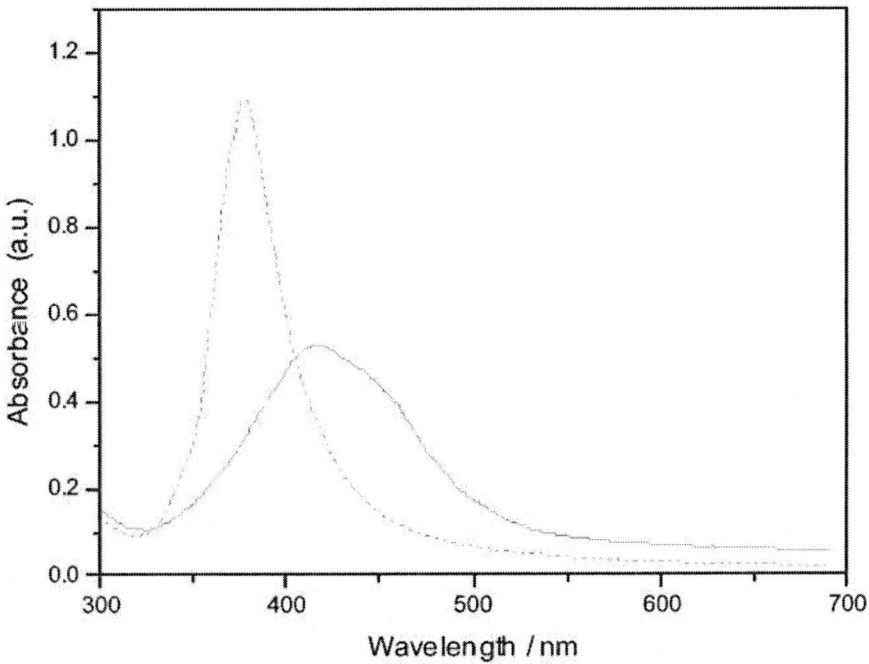

Figure 3. Absorption spectra of as-prepared silver colloid (dashed line) in water and PVA-Ag nanocomposite film (solid line) with 0.33 wt % of Ag, Reprinted with permission from Chem. Mater., 2003, 15 (26), pp 5019–5024, Copyright (2003) American Chemical Society."

Mbhele (2003) prepared PVA-Ag nanocomposites, optical studies suggested that a broad surface plasmon absorption band was found at 420 nm wavelength in PVA-Ag nanocomposite films while in pure form it was found at 380 nm revealed Ag nanoparticles embedded in PVA matrixes. The water vapor permeability of poly(vinyl alcohol)/Na^+ montmorillonite nanocomposites was measured, figure 4, and found that the improvement in the water permeability instigates from the boosted modulus of the PVA matrix in the nanocomposites (Strawhecker and Manias 2000).

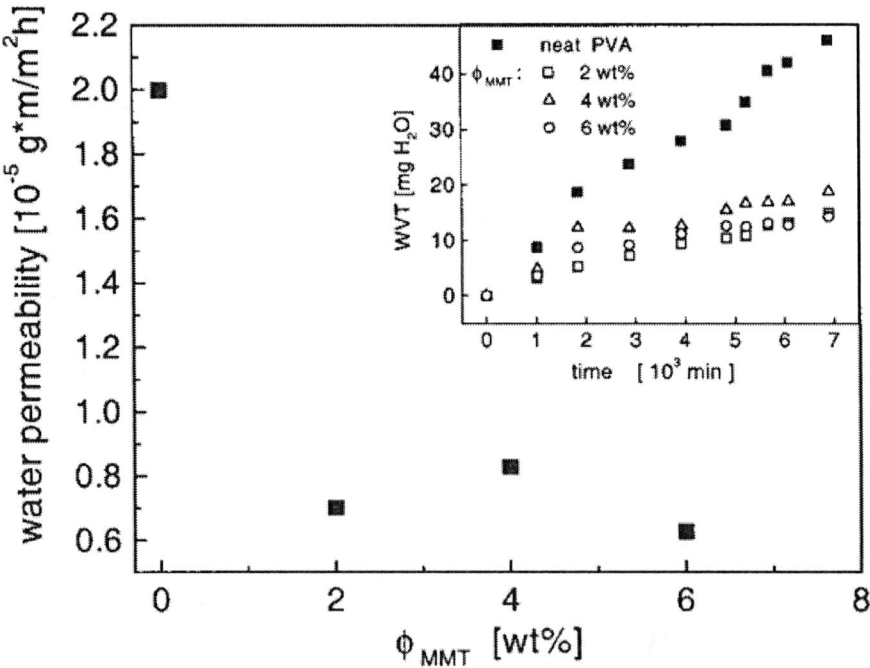

Figure 4. Water vapor permeability for the neat PVA and several PVA/MMT nanocomposites. The inset shows the water vapor transmission raw data collected for each composition, which were used to calculate the water permeabilities. Reprinted with permission from Chem. Mater., 2000, 12 (10), pp. 2943–2949 Copyright (2000) American Chemical Society.

GO/PVA composite hydrogel with enhanced mechanical properties via solution mixing and freezing/thawing was prepared (J. Liu et al., 2012) and unveiled that in PVA chains strong physical cross-linking effect was observed due to hydrogen bonding.

3. Applications

PVA has been used for its compatibility in biomedical applications (Paradossi et al., 2003). Nanocomposites of PVA are used in various biomedical fields like manufacturing of artificial heart surgery contact lenses, wound dressings and drug delivery systems as it has highly favorable properties like biocompatibility, non-carcinogenic, nontoxicity, bioadhesive properties, and swelling characteristics. Polyvinyl alcohol (PVA) reinforced with multi-walled carbon nanotubes and glutaraldehyde is excellent to be used as biomedical applications in an alternative of traditional materials (Mohammad Mahdi Dadfar, Kavoosi, and Mohammad Ali Dadfar 2014).

DRUG DELIVERY SYSTEM AND CANCER DIAGNOSIS

Polyvinyl alcohol and SPION nanocomposites were found useful in drug delivery of popular drug ciprofloxacin [30]. Li, Wang, and Wu (1998) prepared poly(vinyl alcohol) (PVA) hydrogel nanoparticles by the technology of water-in-oil emulsion plus the process of cyclic freezing-thawing for their use in protein (Bovine Serum Albumin)/peptide drug delivery and release of BSA followed diffusion-controlled mechanism. Polyvinyl alcohol (PVA)/halloysite (HNTs) bionanocomposite films were fabricated by solution casting and crosslinking of glutaraldehyde (GA). They exhibited applications in drug delivery systems as well as bone tissue engineering (W. Y. Zhou et al., 2010). PVA-coated indomethacin-loaded PLGA nanocomposites were prepared with an about 100 nm diameter size by emulsification and the solvent evaporation method for their application in iontophoretic transdermal drug delivery (Tomoda et al., 2014). Kalia (2014) reviewed super magnetic iron oxide nanoparticles with PVA in magnetic resonance imaging (MRI) of cancer cells for cancer diagnosis and chemotherapy.

TISSUE ENGINEERING

Nowadays, bone tissue engineering has become one of the auspicious areas because it has the potential to repair diseased/damaged bone tissue by joining osteogenic cells, osteoconductive scaffolds and osteoinductive biological signals organized in an arranged way for bone tissue regeneration (Hou et al., 2007; Bártolo et al., 2009). In order to applications in tissue engineering, Sionkowska and Kozłowska (2010) suggested that nanocomposites processed from collagen type I and PVA showed morphological characteristics for potential use as bone TE soft scaffolds. Polyvinyl alcohol (PVA)/ waterborne polyurethane (WPU)/ TEMPO-oxidized cellulose nanofibers (TOCNs) nanocomposite were prepared (Dai et al., 2014) and they were non-toxic, hydrophilic and biocompatible so could be used for filtration materials, tissue scaffolding and medical fields as wound dressing materials. *Yoshii* and coworkers prepared polyvinyl alcohol (PVA) hydrogel by electron beam irradiation and acetalization of PVA. Heat resistance of these was checked by mechanical properties. Its application as a wound dressing was assessed by attributing to a wound or burn of the back skin of marmots and found homogeneous adhesion to the infected parts along with easy removal with no damage to rehabilitated skin as well as a little rapid rate of regeneration of the injured skin (Yoshii et al., 1995). In the series fabrication of polyvinyl alcohol (PVA) scaffold for bone tissue engineering via selective laser sintering was done by *Shuai and coworkers* (Shuai et al., 2013). They suggested that the porosity of the above was found $67.9 \pm 2.7\%$ which was suitable for the prerequisite of micro-pores of the bone scaffolds as tissue engineering (TE). For wound dressing on animals, nanocomposites of polyvinyl alcohol (PVA) with organically-modified montmorillonite as nano clay was prepared by the freezing-thawing cyclic method. In vivo studies of these were performed which unveiled an enhanced healing process in wounds as compare to sterile gauze and in vitro studies helped to determine cytotoxicity and biocompatibility of synthesized nanocomposites. In studies, these were found non-toxic and biocompatible for their use in wound dressing in practical wound management (Mohammad Sirousazar, Kokabi, and Hassan 2011). Preparation of nanocomposites of polyvinyl alcohol- chitosan (PVA-CS) and graphene oxide (GO) was done by casting their stable aqueous mixture. These new nanocomposites revealed enhanced thermal stability as well as they were found mechanically strong. Their cell viability and cytotoxicity studies unveiled that MC3T3-E1 mouse osteoblastic cells can attach and fabricated on PVA-CS/GO nanocomposite films and makes them a suitable candidate for tissue engineering (Pandele et al., 2014). Nanocomposites of

PVA and chitosan prepared by gamma radiations revealed good biodegradability, biocompatibility, and hemostatic properties and due to this, they can be used in wound dressing (El Salmawi 2007).

OTHER BIOMEDICAL APPLICATIONS

Polyvinyl alcohol (PVA) functionalized cobalt ferrite nanocomposites were successfully prepared by the combustion method and surface modified by (Salunkhe et al., 2013) for biomedical applications. These were characterized by X-ray diffraction (XRD), transmission electron microscopy (TEM), Fourier transforms infrared (FTIR) spectroscopy, dynamic light scattering (DLS) and thermogravimetric analysis (TGA) and revealed decrement of contact angle suggested the conversion of hydrophobic nature to hydrophilic. In vitro cytotoxicity results revealed less cytotoxicity of these on mouse fibroblast L929 cell line. A novel nanocomposite polyvinyl alcohol/polyaniline/ Ag (PVA/PANI/Ag) was developed by exposure of Ag nanoparticles on the PVA/PANI composite. These nanocomposites showed outstanding antibacterial activity against Gram-positive bacteria *Staphylococcus aureus* and Gram-negative *Escherichia coli* with the help of a paper disk diffusion method (Ghaffari-Moghaddam and Eslahi 2014). Nanoparticles of $Zn_{0.5}Co_{0.5}Al_{0.5}Fe_{1.46}La_{0.04}O_4$ remove dye up to 76% while the $Zn_{0.5}Co_{0.5}Al_{0.5}Fe_{1.46}La_{0.04}O_4$/PVA nanocomposites removed the dye up to 90% suggested its potential application in industrial wastewater purifying and recycling (Ahmed et al., 2013).

CONCLUSION

Over the past few decades, polymeric nanocomposites are in high demand due to its unique properties that can be attained with these materials. These nanocomposites revealed a wide and versatile range of properties and other beneficial characteristics at adequate cost and biodegradation rate, thus can be applied in a broad range of applications. The alternative polymeric medical devices are popular and have also increased substantially around the world. As a host for different kinds of nanofiller in these nanocomposites, poly(vinyl alcohol) (PVA) plays an important role as it is a water-soluble polymer. The introduction of nanosized particles into the PVA enhanced its properties and makes it an outstanding tool for biomedical uses. This chapter provides an overview of recent advances in polyvinyl alcohol (PVA) based nanocomposites and its applications in different medical fields such as drug delivery, wound healing, bone replacement, tissue engineering, and others.

REFERENCES

Ahmed, M A, Rasha M Khafagy, Samiha T Bishay, and N M Saleh. 2013. "Effective Dye Removal and Water Purification Using the Electric and Magnetic Zn0.5Co0.5Al0.5Fe1.46La0.04O4/Polymer Core–shell Nano-composites." *Journal of Alloys and Compounds* 578: 121–31. doi:https://doi.org/10.1016/j.jallcom.2013.04.182.

Bártolo, P J, C K Chua, H A Almeida, S M Chou, and A S C Lim. 2009. "Biomanufacturing for Tissue Engineering: Present and Future Trends." *Virtual and Physical Prototyping* 4 (4). Taylor & Francis: 203–16. doi:10.1080/17452750903476288.

BUNN, C W. 1948. "Crystal Structure of Polyvinyl Alcohol." *Nature* 161 (June). Nature Publishing Group: 929. https://doi.org/10.1038/161929a0.

Dai, Lei, Zhu Long, Xue-hong Ren, Hai-bo Deng, Hong He, and Wen Liu. 2014. "Electrospun Polyvinyl Alcohol/Waterborne Polyurethane Composite Nanofibers Involving Cellulose Nanofibers." *Journal of Applied Polymer Science* 131 (22). John Wiley & Sons, Ltd. doi:10.1002/app.41051.

DeMerlis, C C, and D R Schoneker. 2003. "Review of the Oral Toxicity of Polyvinyl Alcohol (PVA)." *Food and Chemical Toxicology* 41 (3). Elsevier: 319–26.

Feldman, Dorel. 2016. "Polymer Nanocomposites in Medicine." *Journal of Macromolecular Science, Part A* 53 (1). Taylor & Francis: 55–62.

Ghaffari-Moghaddam, Mansour, and Hassan Eslahi. 2014. "Synthesis, Characterization and Antibacterial Properties of a Novel Nanocomposite Based on Polyaniline/Polyvinyl Alcohol/Ag." *Arabian Journal of Chemistry* 7 (5): 846–55. doi:https://doi.org/10.1016/j.arabjc.2013.11.011.

Hill, David J T, and Tri T Le. 2001. "An ESR Study on γ-Irradiated Poly (Vinyl Alcohol)." *Radiation Physics and Chemistry* 62 (2–3). Elsevier: 283–91.

Hou, Lein-Tuan, Cheng-Meei Liu, Bu-Yuan Liu, Po-Chun Chang, Min-Huei Chen, Ming-Hua Ho, Su-Min Jehng, and Hwa-Chang Liu. 2007. "Tissue Engineering Bone Formation in Novel Recombinant Human Bone Morphogenic Protein 2–Atelocollagen Composite Scaffolds." *Journal of Periodontology* 78 (2). John Wiley & Sons, Ltd: 335–43. doi:10.1902/jop.2007.060106.

Hyon, S-H, W-I Cha, and Y Ikada. 1989. "Preparation of Transparent Poly (Vinyl Alcohol) Hydrogel." *Polymer Bulletin* 22 (2). Springer: 119–22.

Jalal Uddin, Ahmed, Jun Araki, and Yasuo Gotoh. 2011. "Toward 'Strong' Green Nanocomposites: Polyvinyl Alcohol Reinforced with Extremely Oriented Cellulose Whiskers." *Biomacromolecules* 12 (3). American Chemical Society: 617–24. doi:10.1021/bm101280f.

Kalia, Susheel, Sarita Kango, Amit Kumar, Yuvaraj Haldorai, Bandna Kumari, and Rajesh Kumar. 2014. "Magnetic Polymer Nanocomposites for Environmental and Biomedical Applications." *Colloid and Polymer Science* 292 (9). Springer: 2025–52.

Lee, Joon Seok, Kyu Ha Choi, Han Do Ghim, Sam Soo Kim, Du Hwan Chun, Hak Yong Kim, and Won Seok Lyoo. 2004. "Role of Molecular Weight of Atactic Poly (Vinyl Alcohol)(PVA) in the Structure and Properties of PVA Nanofabric Prepared by Electrospinning." *Journal of Applied Polymer Science* 93 (4). Wiley Online Library: 1638–46.

Li, Jia Kui, Nuo Wang, and Xue Shen Wu. 1998. "Poly(Vinyl Alcohol) Nanoparticles Prepared by Freezing–thawing Process for Protein/Peptide Drug Delivery." *Journal of Controlled Release* 56 (1): 117–26. doi:https://doi.org/10.1016/S0168-3659(98)00089-3.

Liang, Jiajie, Yi Huang, Long Zhang, Yan Wang, Yanfeng Ma, Tianyin Guo, and Yongsheng Chen. 2009. "Molecular-level Dispersion of Graphene into Poly (Vinyl Alcohol) and Effective Reinforcement of Their Nanocomposites." *Advanced Functional Materials* 19 (14). Wiley Online Library: 2297–2302.

Limpan, Natthaporn, Thummanoon Prodpran, Soottawat Benjakul, and Surasit Prasarpran. 2012. "Influences of Degree of Hydrolysis and Molecular Weight of Poly (Vinyl Alcohol)(PVA) on Properties of Fish Myofibrillar Protein/PVA Blend Films." *Food Hydrocolloids* 29 (1). Elsevier: 226–33.

Liu, Jiaqi, Caifeng Chen, Changcheng He, Jing Zhao, Xiaojing Yang, and Huiliang Wang. 2012. "Synthesis of Graphene Peroxide and Its Application in Fabricating Super Extensible and Highly Resilient Nanocomposite Hydrogels." *ACS Nano* 6 (9). American Chemical Society: 8194–8202. doi:10.1021/nn302874v.

Liu, Mingxian, Baochun Guo, Mingliang Du, and D Jia. 2007. "Drying Induced Aggregation of Halloysite Nanotubes in Polyvinyl Alcohol/Halloysite Nanotubes Solution and Its Effect on Properties of Composite Film." *Applied Physics A* 88 (2). Springer: 391–95.

Mansur, Herman S, Rodrigo L Oréfice, and Alexandra A P Mansur. 2004. "Characterization of Poly (Vinyl Alcohol)/Poly (Ethylene Glycol) Hydrogels and PVA-Derived Hybrids by Small-Angle X-Ray Scattering and FTIR Spectroscopy." *Polymer* 45 (21). Elsevier: 7193–7202.

Mansur, Herman S, Carolina M Sadahira, Adriana N Souza, and Alexandra A P Mansur. 2008. "FTIR Spectroscopy Characterization of Poly (Vinyl Alcohol) Hydrogel with Different Hydrolysis Degree and Chemically Crosslinked with Glutaraldehyde." *Materials Science and Engineering: C* 28 (4). Elsevier: 539–48.

Mbhele, Z. H., Salemane, M. G., CGCE Van Sittert, J M Nedeljković, V Djoković, and A S Luyt. 2003. "Fabrication and Characterization of Silver− Polyvinyl Alcohol Nanocomposites." *Chemistry of Materials* 15 (26). ACS Publications: 5019–24.

Mohammad Mahdi Dadfar, Seyed, Gholamreza Kavoosi, and Seyed Mohammad Ali Dadfar. 2014. "Investigation of Mechanical Properties,

Antibacterial Features, and Water Vapor Permeability of Polyvinyl Alcohol Thin Films Reinforced by Glutaraldehyde and Multiwalled Carbon Nanotube." *Polymer Composites* 35 (9). Wiley Online Library: 1736–43.

Pal, Kunal, Ajit K Banthia, and Dipak K Majumdar. 2007. "Preparation and Characterization of Polyvinyl Alcohol-Gelatin Hydrogel Membranes for Biomedical Applications." *Aaps Pharmscitech* 8 (1). Springer: E142–46.

Pandele, Andreea Madalina, Mariana Ionita, Livia Crica, Sorina Dinescu, Marieta Costache, and Horia Iovu. 2014. "Synthesis, Characterization, and in Vitro Studies of Graphene Oxide/Chitosan–polyvinyl Alcohol Films." *Carbohydrate Polymers* 102: 813–20. doi:https://doi.org/10.1016/j.carbpol.2013.10.085.

Paradossi, Gaio, Francesca Cavalieri, Ester Chiessi, Chiara Spagnoli, and Mary K Cowman. 2003. "Poly (Vinyl Alcohol) as Versatile Biomaterial for Potential Biomedical Applications." *Journal of Materials Science: Materials in Medicine* 14 (8). Springer: 687–91.

Qiu, Kaiyan, and Anil N Netravali. 2012. "Fabrication and Characterization of Biodegradable Composites Based on Microfibrillated Cellulose and Polyvinyl Alcohol." *Composites Science and Technology* 72 (13). Elsevier: 1588–94.

———. 2013. "Halloysite Nanotube Reinforced Biodegradable Nanocomposites Using Noncrosslinked and Malonic Acid Crosslinked Polyvinyl Alcohol." *Polymer Composites* 34 (5). Wiley Online Library: 799–809.

Razzak, Mirzan T, and Darmawan Darwis. 2001. "Irradiation of Polyvinyl Alcohol and Polyvinyl Pyrrolidone Blended Hydrogel for Wound Dressing." *Radiation Physics and Chemistry* 62 (1). Elsevier: 107–13.

Roohani, Mehdi, Youssef Habibi, Naceur M Belgacem, Ghanbar Ebrahim, Ali Naghi Karimi, and Alain Dufresne. 2008. "Cellulose Whiskers Reinforced Polyvinyl Alcohol Copolymers Nanocomposites." *European Polymer Journal* 44 (8). Elsevier: 2489–98.

Salavagione, Horacio J, Marian A Gomez, and Gerardo Martinez. 2009. "Polymeric Modification of Graphene through Esterification of

Graphite Oxide and Poly (Vinyl Alcohol)." *Macromolecules* 42 (17). ACS Publications: 6331–34.

Salmawi, Kariman M El. 2007. "Gamma Radiation-Induced Crosslinked PVA/Chitosan Blends for Wound Dressing." *Journal of Macromolecular Science, Part A* 44 (5). Taylor & Francis: 541–45.

Salunkhe, A B, V M Khot, N D Thorat, M R Phadatare, C I Sathish, D S Dhawale, and S H Pawar. 2013. "Polyvinyl Alcohol Functionalized Cobalt Ferrite Nanoparticles for Biomedical Applications." *Applied Surface Science* 264: 598–604. doi:https://doi.org/10.1016/j.apsusc.2012.10.073.

Shuai, Cijun, Zhongzheng Mao, Haibo Lu, Yi Nie, Huanlong Hu, and Shuping Peng. 2013. "Fabrication of Porous Polyvinyl Alcohol Scaffold for Bone Tissue Engineering via Selective Laser Sintering." *Biofabrication* 5 (1). IOP Publishing: 15014. doi:10.1088/1758-5082/5/1/015014.

Sindhu, S, S Jegadesan, A Parthiban, and S Valiyaveettil. 2006. "Synthesis and Characterization of Ferrite Nanocomposite Spheres from Hydroxylated Polymers." *Journal of Magnetism and Magnetic Materials* 296 (2): 104–13. doi:https://doi.org/10.1016/j.jmmm.2005.02.002.

Sionkowska, Alina, and Justyna Kozłowska. 2010. "Characterization of Collagen/Hydroxyapatite Composite Sponges as a Potential Bone Substitute." *International Journal of Biological Macromolecules* 47 (4): 483–87. doi:https://doi.org/10.1016/j.ijbiomac.2010.07.002.

Sirousazar, M, M Kokabi, Z M Hassan, and A R Bahramian. 2011. "Dehydration Kinetics of Polyvinyl Alcohol Nanocomposite Hydrogels Containing Na-Montmorillonite Nanoclay." *Scientia Iranica* 18 (3). Elsevier: 780–84.

Sirousazar, Mohammad, Mehrdad Kokabi, and Zuhair Muhammad Hassan. 2011. "In Vivo and Cytotoxic Assays of a Poly(Vinyl Alcohol)/Clay Nanocomposite Hydrogel Wound Dressing." *Journal of Biomaterials Science, Polymer Edition* 22 (8). Taylor & Francis: 1023–33. doi:10.1163/092050610X497881.

Spiridon, Iuliana, Maria Cristina Popescu, Ruxanda Bodârlău, and Cornelia Vasile. 2008. "Enzymatic Degradation of Some Nanocomposites of Poly (Vinyl Alcohol) with Starch." *Polymer Degradation and Stability* 93 (10). Elsevier: 1884–90.

Strawhecker, K E, and E Manias. 2000. "Structure and Properties of Poly (Vinyl Alcohol)/Na+ Montmorillonite Nanocomposites." *Chemistry of Materials* 12 (10). ACS Publications: 2943–49.

Tiwari, Ashutosh, Murugan Ramalingam, Hisatoshi Kobayashi, and Anthony P F Turner. 2012. *Biomedical Materials and Diagnostic Devices*. John Wiley & Sons.

Tomoda, Keishiro, Natsumi Yabuki, Hiroshi Terada, and Kimiko Makino. 2014. "Application of Polymeric Nanoparticles Prepared by an Antisolvent Diffusion with Preferential Solvation for Iontophoretic Transdermal Drug Delivery." *Colloid and Polymer Science* 292 (12). Springer: 3195–3203.

Xu, Yuxi, Wenjing Hong, Hua Bai, Chun Li, and Gaoquan Shi. 2009. "Strong and Ductile Poly (Vinyl Alcohol)/Graphene Oxide Composite Films with a Layered Structure." *Carbon* 47 (15). Elsevier: 3538–43.

Yoshii, F, K Makuuchi, D Darwis, T Iriawan, M T Razzak, and Janusz M Rosiak. 1995. "Heat Resistance Poly(Vinyl Alcohol) Hydrogel." *Radiation Physics and Chemistry* 46 (2): 169–74. doi:https://doi.org/10.1016/0969-806X(95)00008-L.

Zhang, Chunxue, Xiaoyan Yuan, Lili Wu, Yue Han, and Jing Sheng. 2005. "Study on Morphology of Electrospun Poly (Vinyl Alcohol) Mats." *European Polymer Journal* 41 (3). Elsevier: 423–32.

Zhang, Xiefei, Tao Liu, T V Sreekumar, Satish Kumar, Valerie C Moore, Robert H Hauge, and Richard E Smalley. 2003. "Poly (Vinyl Alcohol)/SWNT Composite Film." *Nano Letters* 3 (9). ACS Publications: 1285–88.

Zhou, Keqing, Saihua Jiang, Chenlu Bao, Lei Song, Bibo Wang, Gang Tang, Yuan Hu, and Zhou Gui. 2012a. "Preparation of Poly(Vinyl Alcohol) Nanocomposites with Molybdenum Disulfide (MoS2): Structural Characteristics and Markedly Enhanced Properties." *RSC Advances* 2

(31). The Royal Society of Chemistry: 11695–703. doi:10.1039/C2RA21719H.

———. 2012b. "Preparation of Poly (Vinyl Alcohol) Nanocomposites with Molybdenum Disulfide (MoS 2): Structural Characteristics and Markedly Enhanced Properties." *Rsc Advances* 2 (31). Royal Society of Chemistry: 11695–703.

Zhou, Wen You, Baochun Guo, Mingxian Liu, Ruijuan Liao, A Bakr M Rabie, and Demin Jia. 2010. "Poly(Vinyl Alcohol)/Halloysite Nanotubes Bionanocomposite Films: Properties and in Vitro Osteoblasts and Fibroblasts Response." *Journal of Biomedical Materials Research Part A* 93A (4). John Wiley & Sons, Ltd: 1574–87. doi:10.1002/jbm.a.32656.

In: Biocomposites in Bio-Medicine
Editors: Mudasir Ahmad et al.
ISBN: 978-1-53616-247-9
© 2019 Nova Science Publishers, Inc.

Chapter 7

BIOPOLYMERS AND THEIR ROLE IN BIOMEDICINE

Javeed A Ganaie[1,*], *Mudasir Ahmad*[2] *and Baoliang Zhang*[2]

[1]Department of Chemistry, Jiwaji University Gwalior, India
[2]School of Natural and Applied Sciences Northwestern Polytechnical University Xi'an, China

ABSTRACT

Biopolymers are obtained from biowastes or natural origin from various sources used for various industrial applications such as wastewater treatment, photocatalysis, and biomedical applications. Various types of biopolymers are available for biomedical applications due to their inherent properties like antimicrobial activity, biocompatibility, biodegradability. Biopolymers play a vital role in the medical field due to presence of the various functional groups. These functional groups are easy to modify for various applications such as drug delivery, wound healing, and tissue engineering.

---

* Corresponding Author's Email: ganaiejaveed13@gmail.com.

Keywords: biopolymer, classification PLA, chitosan

INTRODUCTION

Biopolymers derived from natural resources are renewable, biodegradable and non-toxic in nature. These polymers are also produced from biological diversity such as plants, animals, and microorganisms. These biopolymers are also synthesized chemically from biological materials such as sugars, starch, natural fats, etc. The use of polymers in medical applications has been used from ancient times. These polymers offered a good design for the materials to make it more biocompatible. In recent years the biological functions of polysaccharides attain a great biomedical application. There are a number of applications of the biopolymers including the food additives, clothing fabrics, water treatment chemicals, packaging of medical materials. There are basically three types of biopolymers which include polysaccharides, proteins, and polynucleotides. The use of the biopolymers in the development of therapeutic devices such as three dimensional porous structures as scaffolds for tissue engineering, controlled release drug delivery and applications like suturing, fixation or adhesion which are developed from the biopolymers whose degradation products are not immunogenic (Niaounakis . 2015, Onar.2014, Reddy et al. 2015). The biopolymers are basically alternative to petroleum-based polymers and their properties depend on the polymer structure.

CLASSIFICATION OF BIOPOLYMERS

The three main groups of the biopolymers are classified in Table 1 on the basis of their origin.

BIOPOLYMERS FOR BIOLOGICAL APPLICATION

Polylactic Acid (PLA)

It is a biopolymer that can be produced from natural sources such as corn starch, potatoes. It can be made into consumer items as diverse as disposable plates and cups, packaging and clothing and some properties of PLA are similar to that of synthetic polymers (Mukherjee et al. 2011). The monomers used for polymerization of lactides are synthesized from glycolic acid, DL lactic acid. PLA (Polylactic acid) comes from fermented plant starch (mostly from corn) and is often referred to as corn starch plastic. It is becoming popular very quickly because corn-based plastic is a more environmentally-friendly alternative to traditional plastics, which are petroleum-based. There are two methods for manufacturing polylactic acid (PLA) from lactic acid: the first method uses the cyclic lactic acid dimer called lactide as an intermediate stage; the second method is direct polymerization of lactic acid. Polylactic acid is formed from the corn which is first fermented to the lactic acid, the lactic acid is then polymerized to make polylactic acid. It is the first bio-plastic which is still used today, these bio-plastics make many contributions to the reduction of CO_2 in the environment and these are also biodegradable substances by which it protects the environment. The bio-plastic materials are used in automobile interiors, for packaging of food items, for agriculture sheeting and other household appliances (Auras et al., 2010, Benninga 1990, Xiao et al. 2012).

Advantages of Corn

(a) Comes from corn, which is a renewable resource
(b) Does not contain toxins
(c) Producing this kind of plastic creates much less greenhouse gas emissions than conventional plastic production.
(d) Less energy is needed to produce corn-based plastic than to produce conventional plastics.

(e) Polylactic acid is more competitive than conventional plastic in terms of cost.

(f) Polylactic acid is safer since there is no danger of explosions in its production.

Table 1. shows the classification of various biopolymers

Classification	Origin	Biopolymers
Polysaccharides	Plant/algal	Starch, Cellulose, Alginate, Carrageenan, Pectin, Konjac
	Animal Bacterial	Chitosan, Hyaluronic acid
	Fungal	Pullulan, Elsnan, Yeast, glucans
	Lipids/Surfactants	Acetoglycerides, waxes, surfactants, Emulsion, Elastin, Resin, Adhesives
Proteins		Wheat gluten, casein, serum albumin
Polyesters		Polyhydroxyalkanoates, polylactic acid
Specialty Polymers		Shellac, Poly-gamma glutamic acid, natural rubber, nylon from castor oil

Chitosan

Chitosan is a cationic polysaccharide (Figure 1) found in the exoskeleton of crustaceans which is produced by deacetylation of chitin by obtaining from the alkalizing process at high temperature. It is a biodegradable polymer, used in different forms and have various applications in industrial and biomedical areas. The important application of the chitosan is in the cell attachment and cell growth and skin regeneration (Balan et al. 2014) used a coating of chitosan and heparin and in order to increase the mechanical properties and acceleration of re-endothelization and the healing process [Meng et al. 2009]. Chen (2009) developed a polymeric stent that is made from chitosan-based films fixed by genipin due to its high oxygen permeability chitosan is used as a material for contact and intraocular lenses[Chen et al.2009].

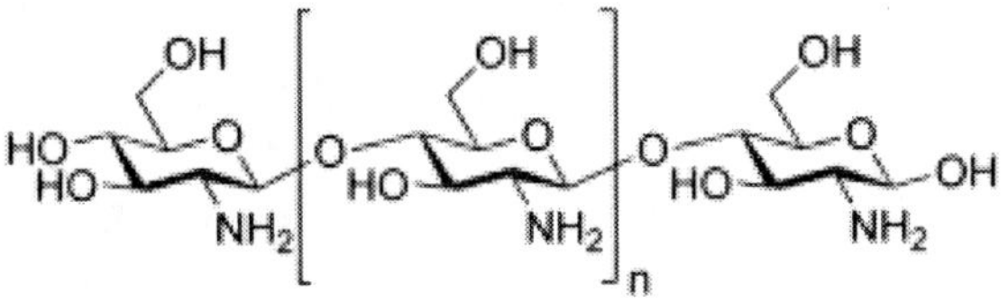

Figure 1. Chemical structure of chitosan (Ahmed et al. 2015, Ahmed et al. 2016).

Biological Properties of Chitosan
- Act as biocompatible (Biodegradable, safe and non-toxic)
- Haemostatic
- Spermicidal
- Antitumor
- Accelerate bone formation
- Central nervous system
- Fungistatic
- Anticholesteremic
- Immunoadjvant.

Application
- Tissue engineering
- Cosmetics
- Ophthalmology
- Artificial Skin
- Wound dressing
- Drug delivery.

Calcium Alginate Biopolymer

This biopolymer is water-soluble, gelatinous and cream-colored substance that can be made by the addition of calcium chloride to the aqueous sodium alginate and gives the artificial flavor and the colors create a tastier edible slime. Calcium alginate is also used in forming the artificial seeds in plant tissue culture. The cell wall of the brown algae is composed of the alginate biopolymer in the sodium salt form of alginic acid (Figure 2).

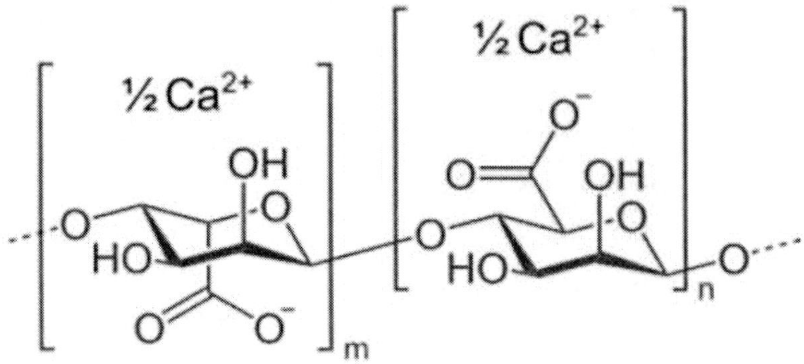

Figure 2. Chemical structure of calcium alginate (https://en.wikipedia.org/wiki/Calcium_alginate).

Applications of Calcium Alginate
   a. For producing the insoluble artificial seeds.
   b. For immobilizing enzymes
   c. To produce an edible substance
   d. Incorporated into wound healing

Collagen and Gelatin

Collagen protein is mostly found in connective tissues and beneath the skin. These proteins present in animals are generally hard and become soft when cooked and it breaks into gelatin which is called cooked collagen, which provides an effective way of absorbing the collagen-boosting amino acids. Gelatin and hydrolyzed collagen which is made from animal collagen and has same profile of amino acid. Some differences in their structure and properties are:

- Hydrolyzed collagen is broken down into smaller units of protein which are easy to digest.
- Hydrolyzed collagen dissolves in both hot and cold water but gelatin does not dissolve.
- Gels of Gelatin can be prepared, but hydrolyzed collagen gels cannot be prepared.

Functional Properties of Collagen and Gelatin
   a. The gelling properties that are associated with collagen and gelatin include gel formation, texturing and water-binding capacity.
   b. The properties related to the surface behavior (emulsion, foam formation, stabilization, adhesion, cohesion, and film-forming capacity) are possibilities of fish collagen as a functional material.

Biological Applications

- The collagen sheets are non-inflammatory and facilitate the migration of fibroblasts and microvascular cells.
- They have low antigenicity and have minimal biodegradation.
- They are non-toxic and helps in minimizing scarring.

CONCLUSION

Biopolymers are an important class of materials that have important applications. Of all these medical applications is an important one. The importance of new medical textiles biopolymers increased day by day due to its versatility, biocompatibility and non-cytotoxicity make these materials excellent for use. New types of polymers like polylactic acid, collagen, chitin, and such others have been used in today's technological period.

REFERENCES

Ahmed S., Ahmad M., Jayachandran M., Qureshi M. A, Ikram S. 2015 Chitosan Based Dressings for Wound Care, *Immunochem Immunopathol*, Volume 1, Issue 2, 1000106.

Ahmed S., Ahmad M., Jayachandran M., Qureshi M. A, Ikram S. 2016 Physicochemical Characterization of Glutaraldehyde Crosslinked Chitosan-Gelatin Films, *Materials Focus*, 5, 1–6.

Auras R., Lim L., Selke S., Tsuji H. 2010 Poly (Lactic Acid): Synthesis, Structures, Properties, Processing, and Applications. *Wiley Online Library*, USA.

Balan V., Verestiuc L. 2014 Strategies to improve chitosan hemocompatibility : A review, *J. Eur. Polym.* 53, 171–188.

Benninga H. 1990 A History of Lactic Acid Making. Kluwer Academic Publishers, Dordrecht.

Chen M., Liu C., Tsai H., Lai W., Chang Y., Sung H. 2009 Mechanical properties, drug eluting characteristics and in vivo performance of a genipin-crosslinked chitosan polymeric stent, *Biomaterials*. 30, 5560-5571. https://en.wikipedia.org/wiki/Calcium_alginate

Meng S., Liu Z., Shen L., Guo Z., Chou L., Zhong W. 2009 The effect of a layer-by-layer chitosan – heparin coating on the endothelialisation and coagulation properties of a coronary stent system, *Biomaterials*. 30, 2276-2283.

Mukherjee T., Kao N. 2011 Biopolymer Reinforced with Natural Fibre: A Review, *J. Polym. Environ.* 19, 714-725.

Niaounakis M. 2015."Biopolymers" Applications and Trends, *Elsevier*.

Onar N. 2014 Usage of Biopolymers in Medical Applications, in: *Proc. 3rd Indo-Czech Text. Res. Conf.*

Reddy N., Reddy R., Jiang Q. 2015 Crosslinking biopolymers for biomedical applications, *Trends Biotechnol.*, 33, 362-369.

Xiao L., Wang B., Yang G., Gauthier M., 2012. Poly (Lactic Acid)-Based Biomaterials: Synthesis, Modification and Applications. *Biomedical Science, Engineering and Technology*: 11.

In: Biocomposites in Bio-Medicine
Editors: Mudasir Ahmad et al.

ISBN: 978-1-53616-247-9
© 2019 Nova Science Publishers, Inc.

Chapter 8

LIGNIN: A WONDERFUL BIOPOLYMER

Bilal A. Bhat[1], and Gulzar Rafiqi[2]*

[1]Department of Chemistry, Govt Degree College Shopian (192303) Kmr India
[2]Department of Chemistry, IUST Awantipora (192122) Kmr India

ABSTRACT

Many years of cumulative research has been conducted on the usage of fiber-reinforced composites for biological, environmental and biomedical applications. For potential applications, full advantage must be taken of the material properties and the manufacturing techniques The three main areas have been addressed and discussed. First, a comprehensive and comparative survey of biocomposites from the existing literature obtained from various sources and their importance in various medical fields has been presented. Second, mechanical designs, manufacturing and exploring aspects of various fibrous polymer matrix composites are explained and described. The third area concern over examples of the design, development, and use of several medical devices and implants using polymer composites. However, being renewable, cheap, recyclable, and biodegradable, they have witnessed rapidly growing interested and attention in terms of industrial, biological, environmental and fundamental applications. So keep the whole in view, the present

---

* Corresponding Author's Email: Barbilal20@gmail.com.

chapter focuses on fiber-based polymer lignin applied to biomedical and environmental applications and presents a comprehensive survey of lignin from the existing literature and its various biomedical and environmental applications. This chapter is the first of its kind to present all the contents together related to lignin that are generally limited to their fundamentals, different methods of synthesis and applications. Lignin is a class of complex organic polymers that form important and vast structural materials in the support tissues of vascular plants and some algae. Lignins are particularly important in the formation of cell walls especially in wood and bark because they lend rigidity and support and do not rot easily. Chemically, lignin is a cross-linked polymer with molecular masses in excess of 10,000 u. It is relatively hydrophobic and rich in aromatic subunits. The degree of polymerization is difficult to measure since the material is heterogeneous in nature. Different types of lignin have been described depending on the means of isolation and structure.

Keywords: biocomposites, biomedical, lignin, biodegradable, polymer

1. INTRODUCTION

Wood is composed of many chemical components, primarily extractives, carbohydrates, and lignin, which are distributed non-uniformly as the result of the anatomical structure of plants and trees. The term lignin is derived from the Latin word Lignum which means wood (De Candolle et al. 1821). Lignin is a complex organic polymer that forms a significant structural material in the support tissues of vascular plants and is one of the most abundant organic polymers on Earth after cellulose. The cellulose walls of the wood become impregnated with lignin. It greatly increases the strength and hardness of the cell and imparts necessary rigidity to the tree. This is essential to woody plants in order that they stand erect (Rouhi et al. 2001). Out of all polymers found in plant cell walls, lignin is the only one that is not composed of carbohydrate (sugar) monomers. In recent years, because of the application of modern methods and availability of techniques and instruments for chemical analysis, the lignin field has developed dramatically. Natural lignin is an amorphous, irregular, random and three-dimensional network of cross-linked co-polymer that containing both aromatic and aliphatic entities (Norstrom 2012). Since the knowledge of lignin has evolved over one hundred years and the importance of lignin has been widely recognized since the early 1900s (Glasser et al. 2000). But however, our understanding of lignin is still limited due to its complex structure. Lignins are highly functionalized biomacromolecules possessing primarily alkyl-aryl ether linkages, aliphatic and aromatic hydroxyl groups and low polydispersity, which offer the potential for higher value-added applications in renewable polymeric materials development. About two-thirds of the lignin bonds are of ether type and about one-third is carbon-carbon linkages but the most common linkage is the ß-o-4' linkage which is susceptible to pulping and bleaching and biodegrading reactions whereas the covalent carbon-carbon bonds are more stable (Sjortrom 1993). That is why it is undesirable in most chemical papermaking fibers and is removed by pulping and bleaching processes easily.

1.1. Source

Lignin is a natural resin that fills spaces between plant cells and strengthens cell walls by covering cellulose micro-fibrils. So, it is the main component of plant biomass including cellulose and hemicelluloses. Hence, it can be derived from various sources such as cereal straws, bamboo, bagasse, and wood. In terms of weight, the lignin content in wood is the highest (20 – 35%) while only 3 – 25% in other sources (Smolarski 2012).

1.2. Composition and Structure

Lignin is an amorphous, random and three-dimensional network of cross-linked copolymer of long chains of different types of phenyl propane monomers (lignols) which are considered to be essential lignin precursors (Figure 1). The three main building blocks of lignin preparation are derived from phenylpropane: 4-hydroxy-3-methoxyphenylpropane, 3,5-dimethoxy-4-hydroxyphenylpropane, and 4-hydroxypropane.

These three basic structural monomers include p-phenyl monomer (H type) derived from coumaryl alcohol, guaiacyl monomer (G type) derived from coniferyl alcohol, and syringyl monomer (S type) derived from sinapyl alcohol. The structure of lignin is highly complicated composed of phenylpropane units linked to each other by the irregular coupling of C–C and C–O (Qiu et al. 2006). Ether bonds in lignin include phenol-ether bonds, alkyl-ether bonds, dialkyl, and diaryl ether bonds, and so on. Lignin in softwood and hardwood mainly contains aryl glycerol-β-aryl-(β-O-4) ether bonds. In the C–C bonds of lignin, the dominant coupling type is β-5, β-β linkage, followed by β-1, β-2, 5–5, and so on (Tao et al. 2003). Because the types and positions of functional groups lignins are different with different chemical characteristics.

The polymerization of lignin macromolecules by phenylpropane units is dehydro-oligomerization. The German eminent scientist Freudenberg produced first synthetic lignin by coniferyl alcohol and laccase under aerobic conditions. Later, peroxidase (POD) was found to catalyze this polymerization reaction effectively. In this process, redox shuttles of Mn_3C-Mn_2C played an important role in lignin biosynthesis. There have been several different hypotheses to explain lignification- one is a random coupling model, which proposed that lignol molecules are gradually connected to the lignin polymer by oxidative coupling. The random coupling hypothesis is reasonable because it explains the plasticity of lignin biosynthesis in mutants and transgenesis research. Another hypothesis involves the dirigent-like protein model, which considered that the lignified process is strictly under the manipulation of dirigent-like protein by controlling the formation of particular chemical bonds of the lignin molecules. The hypothesis showed that the metabolism of lignin should be an orderly life process, which explains the large numbers of O-4 linkages in lignin molecules. The formation of sinapyl alcohol and coniferyl alcohol was a relatively independent process by which enzymes involved in sinapyl alcohol synthesis were associated with each other to form a multienzyme complex. The synthesis of coniferyl alcohol is conducted in the cytoplasm another way. The phenylalanine ammonia-lyase (PAL), caffeoyl CoA methyltransferase (CCOMT), CCR, and CAD distribute in the cytoplasm, catalyzing the synthesis of coniferyl alcohol. Peroxidase is widespread in plants with multiformity. So, how it participates in lignin monomer polymerization needs further studies. So far, it remains uncertain whether the POD or laccase catalyzes the polymerization of lignin monomers in the plant or if they work synergistically (Jiang 2001).

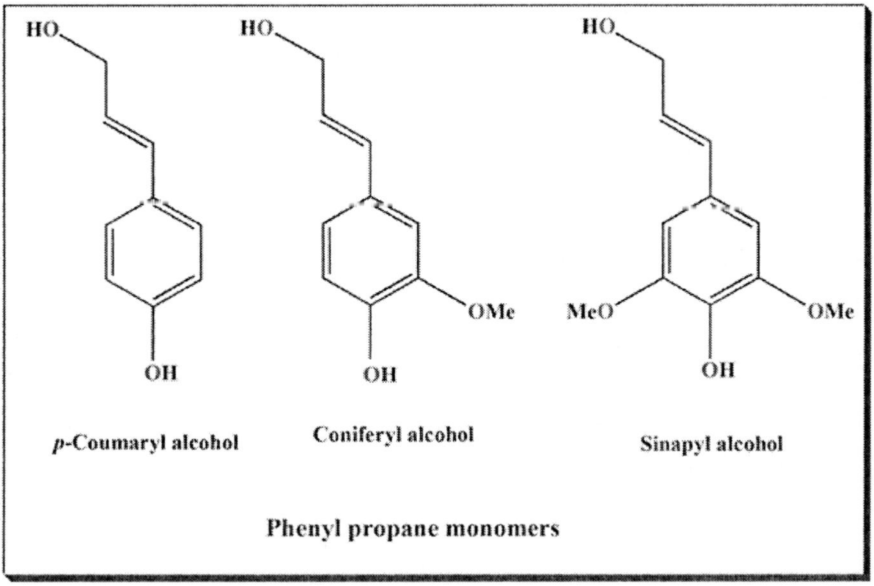

Figure 1. Phenyl propane monomers of lignin.

2. PROPERTIES

The physical, as well as chemical properties of lignin, are revealed as under:

2.1. Physical Properties

The physical properties of the lignin are given as below:

(a) *Molecular weight and polydispersity*
Under the effect of mechanical action, enzymes, or chemical reagents, the three-dimensional net structure of lignin is degraded into different size lignin fragments leads to its molecular weight polydispersity.

(b) *Solubility*
The presence of hydroxyls and many polar groups in the lignin resulting in strong intramolecular and intermolecular hydrogen bonds and making the intrinsic lignin insoluble in any solvent. But however, the presence of phenolic hydroxyl and carboxyl makes the lignin able to be dissolved in alkaline solution.

(c) *Thermal properties*
Lignin is an amorphous thermoplastic polymer. It has slight friability under high temperature and cannot form the film in a solution. It also has glassy transfer properties. The softening temperature of absolutely dried lignin ranges from 127 to 129°C, which remarkably decreased with increased water content, indicating that water acts as a plasticizer in lignin

(d) *Color*
Intrinsic lignin is a white or nearly colorless substance; the color of lignin we can see is the result of the separation and preparation process.

2.2. Chemical Properties

The chemical properties of lignin include nitration, halogenation and oxidation reactions on the phenyl ring of the lignin. It can also undergo benzyl alcohol, the aryl ether bond, and an alkyl ether bond and lignin-modified chromogenic reaction. The chemical reactions of the lignin structural unit are divided into two major categories:

(a) Chemical reactions due to side chain of the lignin
(b) Chemical reaction due to aromatic ring in the lignin structure

(c) Lignin chromogenic reaction

(a) Chemical Reactions Due to Side Chain of the Lignin

Reactions on the lignin side chains are associated with pulping and lignin modification due to nucleophilic reaction. The following reagents can conduct nucleophilic reactions with lignin:

(i) In alkaline medium, the effect of HO^-, HS^-, and S^{-2} nucleophilic reagents leads to the cleavage of the main ether bond, fragmentation and partial dissolution of macromolecule lignin. Hence, the phenol type structural unit is separated into phenolate anions and leads to the activation of *ortho-* and *para-* positions and thereby affects the stability of the CO bond and aryl ether bond is cleaved.

(ii) In a neutral medium, reaction with nucleophile HSO_3^- or SO_3^{2-} leads to breaking of the ether bond and brings and also degradation of lignin fragments.

(iii) In acidic medium, the lignin fragmentation reaction pulping process id carried out. SO_2 aqueous solution leads to the breakage of phenol-type and non-phenolic aryl ether bonds. The sulphonation of carbon may increase the lignin's hydrophilicity. Phenol-type and nonphenolic alkoxy ether bonds may also have a similar type of chemical reaction (Gao et al. 1996; Tao et al. 2003).

(b) Chemical Reaction Due to Aromatic Ring in the Lignin Structure

Chemical reactions of the aromatic ring of lignin are closely related to the lignin-bleaching process and have been divided into electrophilic and nucleophilic reactions:

(i) Electrophilic substitution reaction: Electrophilic reagents include chlorine, chlorine dioxide, oxygen molecule, ozone, nitro cation, nitroso cation, and so on. The electrophilic reagent replacement breaks the side chains of lignin and leads to the oxidative cleavage of "-aryl ether linkages. The aliphatic side chain is oxidized into a carboxylic acid and the aromatic ring is oxidized into the compound of the o-quinone structure, which will finally be oxidized into dicarboxylic acid derivatives.

(ii) Nucleophilic reaction: Nucleophilic reagents that can react with the aromatic ring of lignin include hydroxide ions, hypochlorite ions, and hydrogen peroxide ions. These nucleophilic reagents can react with the chromophoric groups in the degraded lignin fragments, breaking the chromophoric structure to some extent.

(c) Lignin Chromogenic Reaction

The lignin can undergo the formation of a colored compound by the treatment of different types reagents revealed and discuss as under:

(i) **Mäule chromogenic reaction:** When the Hardwood lignin is treated with $KMnO_4$ and HCl and then ammonia, reddish-violet color is obtained. This is because of the syringyl ring of lignin which generates methoxy o-dihydroxybenzene under the treatment of KMnO4 and HCl. A purple methoxy-o-quinone is obtained after ammonia treatment.

(ii) **Cross-Bevan reaction:** Timber without extractives is treated with chlorine in the wet state; the lignin present will be converted into chlorinated lignin. After sulphonic acid and sodium sulfite treatment, the lignin of hardwood turns into red-purple (Jiang 2001).

3. Chemical Analysis of Lignin

The conventional method for lignin quantitation in the pulp industry is the Klason lignin and acid-soluble lignin test, which is standardized according to TAPPI or NREL(Sluiter et al. 2008) procedure. According to the procedure, The cellulose is first recrystallized and partially depolymerized into oligomers by keeping the sample in 72% sulfuric acid at 30 C for 1 h.

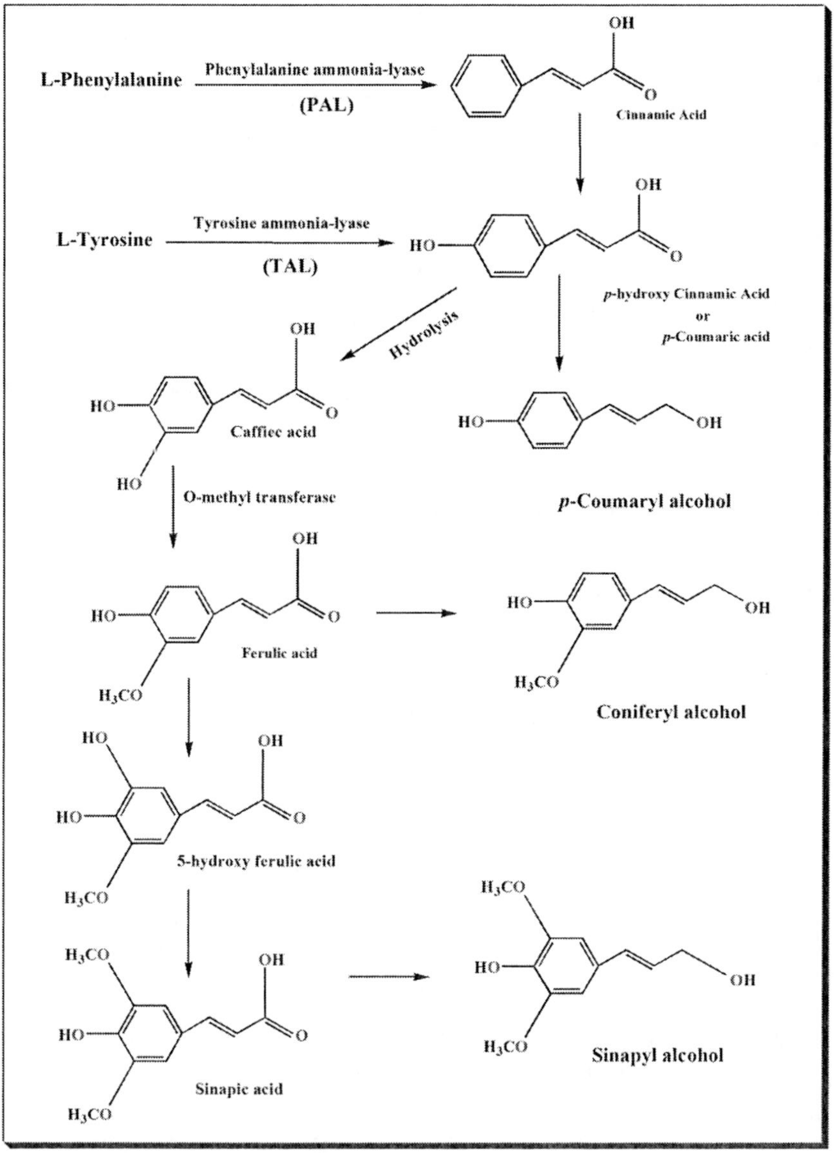

Figure 2. General biosynthesis pathway of monomers of lignin.

Then, the acid is diluted to 4% by adding water, and the depolymerization is completed by either boiling (100°C) for 4 h or pressure cooking at 2 bar (124°C) for 1 h. The acid is washed out and the sample dried. The residue that remains is termed Klason lignin. A part of the lignin, acid-soluble lignin (ASL) dissolves in the acid. ASL is quantified by the intensity of its UV absorption peak at 280 nm. The method is suited for wood lignins, but not equally well for varied lignins from different sources. The carbohydrate composition may be also analyzed from the Klason liquors, although there may be sugar breakdown products (furfural and 5-hydroxymethylfurfural).

A solution of hydrochloric acid and phloroglucinol is used for the detection of lignin (Wiesner test). A brilliant red color develops, owing to the presence of coniferaldehyde groups in the lignin (John 1966).

Thermochemolysis (chemical break down of a substance under vacuum and at high temperature) with tetramethylammonium hydroxide (TMAH) has also been used to analyze the ratios of lignols with fungal decay as well the ratio of the carboxylic acid to aldehyde forms of the lignols. Increases in the lignol value indicate an oxidative cleavage reaction has occurred on the alkyl lignin side chain which has been shown to be a step in the decay of wood by many white-rot and some soft rot fungi.

Solid-state ^{13}C NMR has been used to observe at the concentrations of lignin as well as other major components in wood e.g., cellulose and its change with microbial decay. However, many intact lignins have a cross-linked with a very high molar-mass fraction that is difficult to dissolve even for functionalization.

4. BIOSYNTHESIS

Lignin biosynthesis is a very complex network that is divided into three processes: (i) biosynthesis of lignin monomers (Figure 2) (ii) transport and (iii) polymerization. After a series of steps involving methylation, deamination, hydroxylation, and reduction, lignin monomers are produced in cytoplasm and transported to the apoplast. Finally, lignin is generally polymerized with three main types of monolignols like p-coumaryl alcohol, coniferyl alcohol and sinapyl alcohol (Alejandro et al. 2012; Miao et al. 2010; Bonawitz et al. 2010; Liu et al. 2011). After transport, the lignin precursors are polymerized via free radical reaction. The formation of radicals is catalyzed by oxidative enzymes, either H_2O_2-dependent peroxidases or O_2-dependent oxidases/laccases. These enzymes are secreted into the apoplast where they are either soluble or covalently or ionically bound to the cell wall (Blee et al. 2001).

The two amino acids L-Phenylalanine and L-Tyrosine which are widely present in plants are starting materials for the cinnamic acid pathway (Scheme Figure 2). Under the effects of various enzymes, the three monomers of lignin are finally synthesized after a set of chemical reactions, such as deamination, hydroxylation, methylation, reduction (Li et al. 2003; Geng et al. 2003), etc. Cinnamoyl CoA reductase (CCR) catalyzes the first step of the redox reaction of lignin biosynthesis, which may be the rate-limiting step, controlling lignin synthesis and the pathway from which carbon can go into lignin biosynthesis. Cinnamyl alcohol dehydrogenase (CAD) catalyzes the redox reaction of another step in the lignin synthesis process, which may control the reduction of coniferaldehyde. Sinapylalcohol dehydrogenase (SAD), ferulic acid 5-hydroxylase (F5H), and bispecific caffeic acid/5-hydroxyferulic acid O-methyltransferase (COMT) are immuno-localized in cells and tissues that have S lignin. CAD is located in tissues with precipitation of G lignin. It is speculated that the last step of redox reactions of different types of lignin may be passed through different synthetic pathways and catalyzed by different enzymes. C3H can catalyze coumaric acid to caffeic acid. Most research is inclined mainly to support the lignin biosynthesis and COMT can catalyze the methylation of caffeic acid, 5-hydroxyl coniferyl aldehyde, and 5-hydroxyl coniferyl alcohol into ferulic acid, sinapic acid, and sinapic alcohol, respectively (Lin et al. 2003).

4.1. Factors Influencing Lignin Synthesis

Different parts of plants would have different lignin content and composition. For example, the lignin content and structure are significantly different in the node and internode. The node lignin has a higher density than the internode because of the high content of phenolic acids (p-coumaric acid and ferulic acid). In general, it has been observed that the overuse of nitrogen fertilizer will reduce the lignin content and hence stops the lignification of the plant. However, on the other hand, Phosphate fertilizer will greatly increase the lignin content in the cell wall of the plants.

4.2. Regulation of Lignin Biosynthesis

The lignin biosynthesis may be regulated by changing the activities of different enzymes in two main ways. The first way is to regulate the synthesis process of lignin monomers by simply reducing enzyme activities participating in the lignin synthesis, such as CCR, and CAD, and by reducing the lignin content. The second way is to regulate certain particular enzyme activity to influence the composition and chemical structure of lignin. It is generally believed that the degradation of GS lignin, which is composed of guaiacyl monomers and syringyl monomers, is easier than that for G lignin, which is simply composed of guaiacyl monomers.

In the gene regulation of lignin biosynthesis, the search for and separation of biological enzymes for lignin synthesis will be in first priority in the future. The amino acid sequence of zymoprotein is analyzed to obtain the sequence of its messenger RNA (mRNA), which is the coding sequence of the functional genes. Gene transfer can be done by using different methods like Agrobacterium-mediated indirect conversion and the gene gun technique. Antisense technology can be utilized for regulation of forest lignin. First, an oligonucleotide sequence is constructed that is antisense to the lignin synthase; then, the sequence is transferred into plants in direct or indirect ways, and it interacts with genes in plants to influence the translation and reduce the activity of zymoprotein. This is currently the most common and effective transgenic breeding technology in genetic engineering of lignin regulation. Finding and discovering a natural mutant in plants is also an equally effective and direct means.

5. Polymerization of Lignin

Erdman (1930) studied the oxidative dimerization of various phenols in the biogenesis of natural products and reached the conclusion that lignin must be formed α,β-unsaturated C_6C_3 precursors of the coniferyl alcohol monomer through enzymatic dehydrogenation. Freudenberg and co-workers (1940-1970) had also verified the polymerization of precursors to lignin in nature follow the pathway as Erdman revealed and proposed (Figure 3). In their research, they confirmed that One-electron transfer from coniferyl alcohol by enzymatic dehydrogenation yield resonance-stabilized phenoxy radicals as mechanistically shown below:

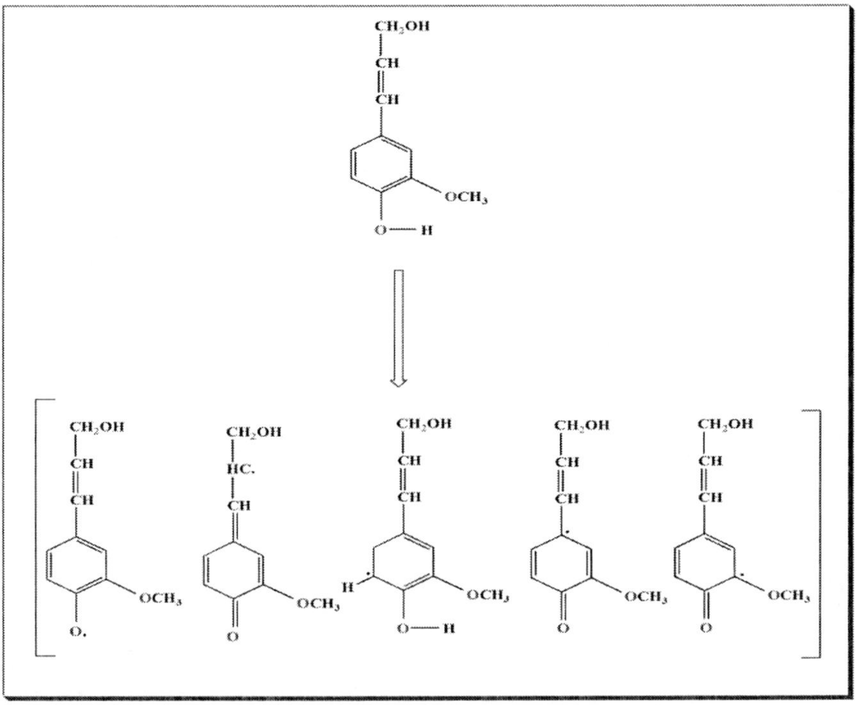

Figure 3. Formation of free radical monomers.

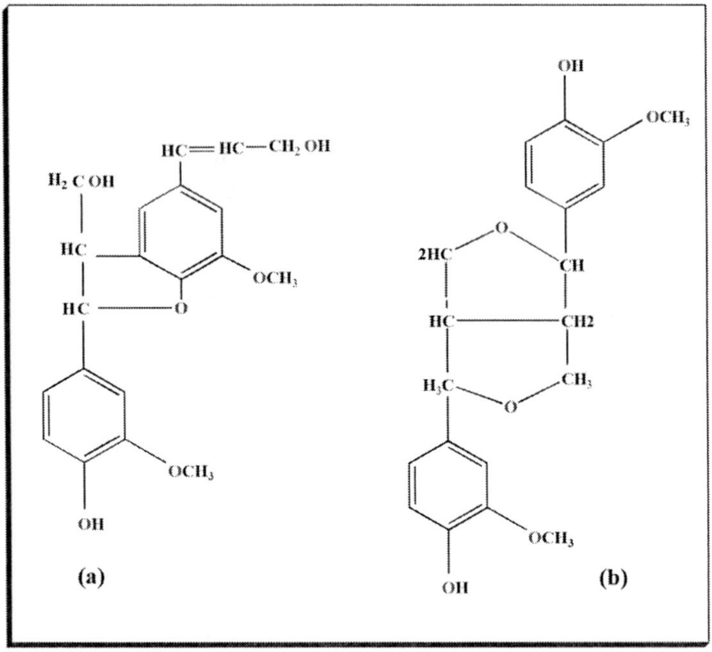

Figure 4. Polymerization of lignin monomer units.

Oligomeric products formed through coupling of coniferyl alcohol radicals as shown above. Endwise β-*O*-4 coupling of a coniferyl alcohol radical with a growing lignin group radical to an intermediate quinone methide (a) which is stabilized to a quaiacylglycerol-β-aryl ether (b) structure through addition of water (Figure 4). The scheme of oligomeric units polymerization is shown as under.

5.1. Types of Linkage and Dimeric Structure

It is clear and proved by the experiments that phenyl propane units are joined together both with C-O-C (ether) and C-C linkages. But however, the C-O-C linkages is dominant and is approximately 2/3 or more in the lignin structure. While the rest of the linkages are C-C type. Proportions of different type of linkages connecting the phenylpropane units in lignin are tabulated as below:

Table 1. Type of linkage and dimer structure

Linkage type	Dimer structure
β-O-4	Aryl glycerol-β-aryl ether
α-O-4	Noncyclic benzyl aryl ether
β-5	Phenylcoumaran
5-5	Biphenyl
4-O-5	Diaryl ether
β-1	1,2-Diaryl propane
β-β	Linkage through side chains

Table 2. Functional groups of lignin (per 100 C_6C_3 units)

Functional group	Softwood lignin	Hardwood lignin
Methoxyl	92 - 97	139 - 158
Phenolic hydroxyl	15 - 30	10 - 15
Benzyl alcohol	30 - 40	40 - 50
Carbonyl	10 - 15	-

5.2. Functional Groups in the Lignin Polymer

Lignin is a polymer contains characteristic Methoxyl groups, phenolic hydroxyl groups, and some terminal aldehyde groups in the side chain. However, only relatively few of the phenolic hydroxyls are free and most of them are occupied through linkages to the neighboring phenylpropane units. The syringyl units in hardwood lignin are extensively etherified. Alcoholic hydroxyl groups and carbonyl groups are introduced into the final lignin polymer during the dehydrogenative polymerization process. In some wood species, substantial amounts of the alcoholic hydroxyl groups are esterified with *p*-hydroxybenzoic acid or *p*-hydroxycinnamic acid. Ester of *p*-hydroxybenzoic acid is typical in aspen lignin. *p*-hydroxycinnamic acid is abundant in bamboo and grass lignin. The different functional groups and their distribution are tabulated as under:

6. Applications

There are a number of applications of lignin in various fields which are discussed as under:

6.1. Antioxidant

Lignin acts as free radical scavengers. It's natural antioxidant properties provide a best use in cosmetic and topical formulations. Lignin sulfonate containing cosmetic compositions have been developed for decorative use on skin.

6.2. Paper

Lignin is used as a sizing agent. The polymerization of acrylamide and hydroxymethylated shown an enhance the tensile strength of paper. Packaging laminate comprising a barrier layer of lignin and oligo or polysaccharides, where the two are partly covalently bonded to each other.

6.3. Agriculture

The slow-release urea is composed of 90 - 99% urea and 1 - 10% lignin. That is why lignin is used either directly or after chemically modified as a binder dispersant agent for pesticides/herbicides, emulsifier and heavy metal sequestrate. The pulverized lignin, when blended with other chemicals, has been used as a soil water retention agent in acidic dry land or desert soil and also as a binder for fertilizer.

6.4. Dispersants

The Dye dispersant is prepared from sulfate or sulfite pulping liquors (lignin) which are cross-linked with formaldehyde products exhibit amazing properties like good dispersion, heat resistant stability, high-temperature dispersion property. Since the lignin sulfonates are biodegradable and non-toxic in nature and hence are used to prepare Jet printing ink. Chemically modified lignin has been used as a dispersing agent, complexing agent, flocculent, thickener or auxiliary agents for coatings, paints or adhesives. A mixture of polycarboxylic acid and lignin sulphonic acid has been used for cleaning aluminum plates.

6.5. Grease

When the calcium lignin sulphonate has been added to grease used to thickened the base grease in order to improve its lubricating quality. The grease which is mixed with lignin had improved not only corrosion protection properties but also provides anti-friction properties with longer lubrication life.

6.6. Heat

Since the artificial firelog using cellulosic matter, nonpetroleum based wax (lignin) and 1,3-propanediol derived from a renewable resource. However when an Indulin based lignin is added to wood pellets produces better quality pellets with high both fuel quality and value.

6.7. Fuel

The alkaline purified lignin, when mixed with diesel, are using as surfactants/emulsifiers. The lignin can be converted into the green gasoline or diesel catalytically (metal precursor such as ruthenium or vanadium and a bidentate ligand) by the combination of different chemical methods pyrolysis, thermal cracking, hydrocracking or hydrocracking.

6.8. Battery

The lignin has great importance in batteries as it forms a thin layer on the graphite powder surface which prevents the battery from decreasing Hydrogen overvoltage and does not affect the condition of the graphite powder. It can also suppress generation of $4PbO.PbSO_4$ compound and hence enhances performance of energy storage devices.

6.9. Concrete

Low levels of lignin and its modified lignin can yield high-performance concrete strength aid. It can reduce damage to building external wall which can be caused by moisture and acid rain. Select lignins can improve the compressive strength of cement pastes and improves its binding property.

6.10. Plastics/Polymers

Lignin based rigid polyurethane resin which is comprised of an epoxy resin and a lignin-derived acid anhydride free lignin known as curing agent used for automotive brakes and epoxy resins for printed circuit boards. Polyphenylene oxide-based polymers and lignin esters are blended to exhibit modulus of elasticity, tensile strength, and elongation at break. Lignin can act as a water absorption inhibitor and as fluidization agents when mixed with polyamide. The use of alkali lignin poly(propylene carbonate) improves thermal stability and mechanical properties of the wonderful polymer.

6.11. Chemicals

One of the best use of lignin is the formations of phenols. Phenols are prepared by reacting lignin with hydrogen supplying solvent at elevated temperature or pressure. The reaction proceeds by the depolymerization of lignin in order to prepare phenolic compounds like:

- Cresols
- Catechols
- Resorcinol
- Quinones
- Vanillin
- Guaiacols

7. FUTURE RESEARCH

In the future, researchers are stressing to replace crude oil by lignin, as it is currently treated as industrial waste. The research route leading to this goal is being paved by new photo-catalysts. Unfortunately, despite many years of attempts by teams of chemists and other researchers from all over the world, still have not managed to develop efficiently. cheaper and successful methods of converting lignin. However, it seems a step closer to cheap solar biorefineries capable of processing lignin on an industrial scale using the new photo-catalysts. On the other hand, the efforts are also focused on how to make more efficient use of major raw materials streams of the paper and pulp industry of lignin. Since the lignin is the natural glue in plants and has a phenolic nature can be proved a new replacement for wood adhesives. An adhesive system for wood composites consisting mainly of lignin will be a new and great achievement in future.

CONCLUSION

The lignin is a wonderful complex natural product, secondary metabolite, and co-polymer. It is the second largest natural product after cellulose. It has a variety of applications in different fields as has been revealed and discussed in detail above. In past and present, a lot of work has been done on lignin. But however, the research on the lignin in future is open and will be a point of interest and consideration because of wood adhesive property of it.

ACKNOWLEDGMENTS

We highly acknowledge Dr. Masood Ayoub Kaloo Assistant professor (Chemistry) GDC Shopian for his discussion and support during various stages of preparation of this chapter. We are also highly thankful to Rukhsana Bilal, Sarhaan Bilal, Miss Gusia, Dr. Rafeeq Bhat and Saba Rafeeq for their valuable guidance and support with respect to the chapter.

REFERENCES

Alejandro, S., Lee, Y., Tohge, T., Sudre, D., Osorio, S., Park, J., Bovet, L., Geldner, N., Fernie, A. R. & Martinoia, E. (2012). "AtABCG29 is a monolignol transporter involved in lignin biosynthesis". *Current Biology*, *22*, 1207-1212.

Bonawitz, N. D. & Chapple, C. (2010). "The genetics of lignin biosynthesis: Connecting genotype to Phenotype". *Annual Review Of Genetics*, *44*, 337-363.

Blee, K. A., Wheatley, E. R., Bonham, V. A., Mitchell, G. P., Robertson, D., Slabas, A. R., Burrell, M. M., Wojtaszek, P. & Bolwell, G. P. (2001). "Proteomic analysis reveals a novel set of cell wall proteins in a transformed tobacco cell culture that synthesises secondary walls as

determined by biochemical and morphological parameters". *Planta*, *212*, 404-415.
De Candolle, A. P. & Sprengel, K. P. J. (1821). "Elements of the philosophy of plants: containing the Principles of scientific botany with a history of the science, and practical illustrations" W. Blackwood, Edinburgh.
Geng, S., Xu, C. S. & Li, Y. C. (2003). "Advance in biosynthesis of lignin and its regulation". *Acta Bot Boreali-Occidentalia Sin*, *23*, 171-181.
Glasser, W. G., Northey, R. A. & Schultz, T. P. (2000). "Lignin: historical, biological, and materials perspective". *American Chimerical Society*. Washington, D C.
Gao, J. & Tang, L. G. (1996). "Cellulose science". Beijing: Science Press, 1-12.
Jiang, T. D. (2001). "*Lignin*" Beijing: Chemical Industry Press, 1-7.
Jiang, T. D. (2001). "*Lignin*". Beijing: Chemical Industry Press.
John, M. H. (1966). "*Lignin production and detection in wood*". U.S. Forest Service Research.
Liu, C. J., Miao, Y. C. & Zhang, K. W. (2011). "Sequestration and transport of lignin monomeric Precursors". *Molecules*, *16*, 710-727.
Li, W., Xiong, J. & Chen, X. Y. (2003). "Advances in the research of physiological significances and genetic regulation of lignin metabolism". *Acta Bot Boreali-Occidentalia Sin*, *23*, 675-681.
Lin, Z. B., Ma, Q. H. & Xu, Y. Y. (2003). "Lignin biosynthesis and its molecular regulation". *Progress in Natural Science*, *13*, 455-461.
Miao, Y. & Liu, C. (2010). "ATP-binding cassette-like transporters are involved in the transport of lignin precursors across plasma and vacuolar membranes". *USA: Proceedings of the National Academy of Sciences*, *107*, 22728–22733.
Nordstrom, Y. (2012). "Development of softwood kraft lignin based carbon fibres". *Licentiate Thesis, Division of Material Science Department of Engineering Sciences and Mathematics*. Lulea University of Technology.
Qiu, W. H. & Chen, H. Z. (2006). "Structure, function and higher value application of lignin". *Journal of Cellulose Science Technology*, *14*, 52–59.

Rouhi, A. M. & Washington, C. (2001). "Only facts will end lignin war". *Science and Technology*, *79*, 52–56.

Sluiter, A., Hames, B., Ruiz, R., Scarlata, C., Sluiter, J., Templeton, D. & Crocker, D. (2008). *"Determination of Structural Carbohydrates and Lignin in Biomass"*. U.S. Department of Energy.

Sjostrom, E. (1993). *"Wood chemistry: fundamentals and application"*. Academic Press: Orlando, 293-298.

Smolarski, N. (2012). *"High-value opportunities for lignin: unlocking its potential"*. Frost & Sullivan.

Tao, Y. Z. & Guan, Y. T. (2003). "Study of chemical composition of lignin and its application". *Journal of Cellulose Science Technology*, *11*, 42–55.

Tao, Y. Z. & Guan, Y. T. (2003). "Study of chemical composition of lignin and its application". *Journal of Cellulose Science Technology*, *11*, 42–55.

ABOUT THE EDITORS

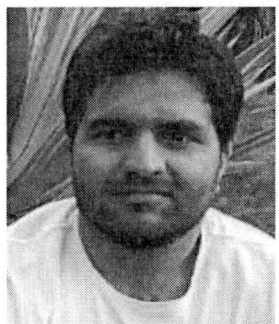

Mudasir Ahmad
Post Doctorate Fellow
School of Natural and Applied Sciences Northwestern
Polytechnical University Xi'an, 710072, PR China
Email: mirmudasirv@gmail.com

Mudasir Ahmad is currently a Post Doc faculty at School of Natural and Applied Sciences NPU, PR China. His current research is focus on Synthesis of Noval Organic/Inorganic Carbon Nanotubes for various industrial applications. In 2018, Mr Ahmad has completed his PhD from the Department of Chemistry Jamia Millia Islamia, New Delhi and worked as SRF fellow from University Grants Commission (UGC) of India. He works closely withseveral programs, State Key Program of National Natural

Science of China (51433008) the National Natural Science China (21704084) and the Fundamental Research Funds for the Central Universities (3102017jc01001). Mr Ahmad has published more than 30papers in reputed journals.

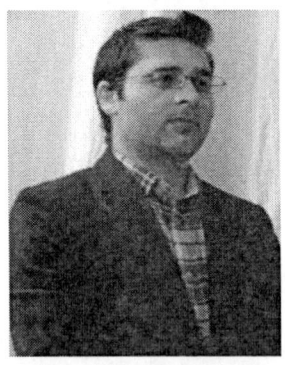

Mohmmad Younus Wani
Assistant Professor
Chemistry Department, Faculty of Sciences, University of Jeddah,
Jeddah, Kingdom of Saudi Arabia
Email: waniyouns@gmail.com

Dr. Wani graduated from Jamia Millia Islamia (Central University), New Delhi, India in 2013. Received a senior research fellowship from CSIR-India in 2012, and FCT postdoctoral fellowship from Portugal in 2013-16.In fall 2016, Dr. Wani moved to the University of Texas, USA and worked with Dr. K. Tsuchikama's group at Texas Therapeutics Institute, Brown Foundation Institute of Molecular Medicine, UTHealth on the development of non-traditional antimicrobial agents and strategies combating multi-drug resistance. Dr. Wani's research interests also include the development of efficient biodegradable materials for biomedical applications. In fall 2017, Dr. Wani was appointed as assistant professor in Chemistry Department, Faculty of Sciences, University of Jeddah, KSA. Dr. Wani continues to work on the development of new molecules and novel strategies to combat microbial infections at the interface of chemistry and biology. He has many international publications, chapters, and Book, besides many international and national honours and awards to his credit.

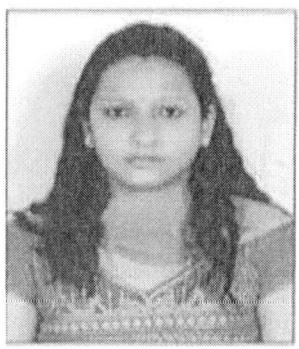

Preeti Singh
Post Doctorate Fellow
Department of Chemistry, Faculty of Natural Sciences,
Jamia Millia Islamia (Central University) New Delhi, India
Email: aries.pre84@gmail.com

Preeti Singh is a Post Doctorate Fellow, UGC in Bio/Polymers Research Laboratory, Department of Chemistry, Jamia Millia Islamia, New Delhi. She was awarded her PhD from the Department of Physics, Faculty of Natural Sciences, Jamia Millia Islamia, New Delhi, India in Physics (Material Science). She has published several research publications in the area of crystal growth and their defects, synthesis of nanomaterials and their applications in Photocatalysis and Sensors. She has authored 23 International Publications along with 3 book chapter and 01 International (edited) book.

About the Editors

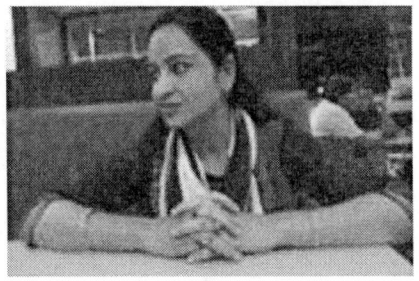

Saiqa Ikram
Associate Professor
Department of Chemistry, Faculty of Natural Sciences,
Jamia Millia Islamia (Central University), New Delhi, Indez
Email: sikram@jmi.ac.in

Saiqa Ikram is working as an Associate Professor, in the Department of Chemistry, Jamia Millia Islamia (A Central University by an Act of Parliament) Delhi, India She is a PhD from Faculty of Technology, University of Delhi followed by Post-doc in Biomedical Engineering from IIT, Delhi. Her pioneering research is in the modification of polymers for sustainable developments. The core polymers are "Chitosan & Cellulose" modified as bio-nanocomposites for therapeutics and compostable materials for wastewater treatment. She had received research funding from Government and Private organizations including Ministry of Science & Technology, Union Grant Commission, Jamia Innovative Research Grant, US-AID & Ministry of Human Resources & Development MHRD-SPARC with University of Queensland, Australia. Under these funding, *"Best Innovative Project Award"* also been felicitated by *US-AID & TERI University in October 2017" (TERI University Research Grant for Innovative Projects)* funded by USAID. These researches brought publications in Journals: Elsevier, Springer, RSC, and ACS, including the book *"Chitosan: Derivatives, Composites & Applications* for *Wiley-Scrivener* -April 2018 & *Biocomposites, Biomedical & Environmental Applications*-November 2017 for *Pan Standford Publishing"*. She had ≥70

International Publications 07 International (edited) book along with ≥13 chapters with other publishers. She had supervised 08 PhD scholars and six more continuing.

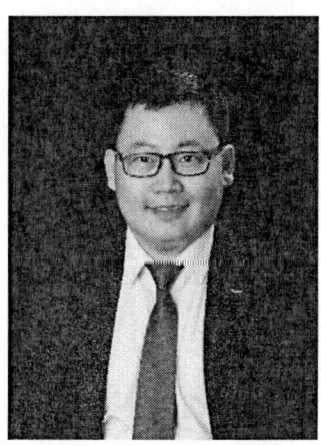

Dr. Baoliang Zhang
Associate Professor
School of Natural and Applied Sciences Northwestern Polytechnical University Xi'an, PR China
Email: blzhang@nwpu.edu.cn

Baoliang Zhang is currently associate professor and doctor student supervisor at Department of Applied Chemistry, NWPU, China. Dr. Zhang received his PhD degree in 2013. He became an assistant professor at Department of Applied Chemistry, NWPU, China in 2014. His research interests focus on: (1) Synthesis and biomedical applications of organic/inorganic magnetic composite microspheres/microcapsules;(2) Modulating mechanism of the impact of porous microspheres on the growth morphology of semiconductors and its environmental applications; (3) Design and applications of protein/phosphate hybrid nanoflowers. He has been in charge of several research subjects, including National Natural Science Foundation of China, the International Cooperation and Exchanges

NSFC, Shaanxi Provincial Natural Science Foundation, Aerospace Science and Technology Innovation Fund. He was awarded the Second Class Prizes of The State Scientific and Technological Progress Award of China as the fourth executer, the Second Prize of Technological Invention Award in Shaanxi province and the First prize of Shaanxi National Defense Science and Technology Advancement Award as the third executer. He has published around 200 research papers and filed more than 50 patents, in which 23 of them were issued.

INDEX

A

anhydro-D-glucopyranose units (AGU), 32
anti-microbial agents, 42
applications, x, 2, 3, 6, 8, 12, 19, 20, 24, 25, 27, 28, 31, 32, 33, 40, 41, 42, 43, 44, 46, 47, 48, 51, 53, 56, 58, 60, 61, 62, 63, 66, 67, 69, 70, 72, 73, 75, 77, 78, 84, 86, 87, 88, 89, 90, 92, 97, 98, 103, 104, 108, 110, 112, 114, 115, 117, 118, 119, 120, 126, 127, 128, 129, 131, 132, 133, 134, 135, 137, 138, 139, 140, 141, 142, 143, 144, 145, 147, 149, 163, 167, 169
artificial grafts, 53, 54

B

biocompatibility, 6, 17, 19, 23, 33, 41, 53, 61, 62, 63, 65, 84, 109, 110, 120, 126, 128, 137, 144
biocomposites, ix, x, 19, 20, 44, 45, 49, 88, 147, 148
biodegradable, ix, 3, 4, 8, 11, 13, 20, 22, 26, 33, 54, 65, 66, 67, 70, 75, 77, 84, 85, 86, 87, 88, 90, 91, 93, 101, 102, 116, 133, 134, 138, 139, 140, 141, 148, 164
biodegradable polymer composites, 33
biomedical, vii, viii, ix, 3, 6, 8, 31, 32, 40, 41, 46, 47, 51, 53, 54, 56, 63, 64, 67, 70, 71, 72, 75, 76, 84, 87, 88, 89, 90, 102, 111, 116, 118, 119, 120, 126, 128, 129, 131, 133, 134, 135, 136, 137, 138, 140, 145, 147, 148
biomedical application, ix, 3, 67, 85, 102, 120, 126, 129, 137, 138, 145, 147
biomedicine, 76, 137
biopolymer(s), ix, 1, 2, 3, 4, 5, 12, 13, 17, 18, 19, 20, 22, 23, 26, 32, 54, 55, 56, 65, 68, 76, 84, 98, 137, 138, 139, 140, 142, 144, 145
bone replacement, 130

C

cellulose, vii, ix, 3, 5, 12, 13, 18, 19, 20, 29, 31, 32, 33, 34, 35, 36, 37, 38, 39, 40, 41, 42, 43, 44, 45, 46, 47, 48, 49, 50, 51, 52, 72, 97, 99, 105, 106, 107, 110, 111, 112, 115, 124, 127, 130, 131, 133, 134, 140, 148, 149, 155, 157, 167, 168, 169
cellulose based nanocomposites, ix, 31, 40, 41

ceramic matrix composites, 33
chitosan, 5, 6, 8, 9, 18, 26, 27, 28, 62, 64, 65, 71, 72, 101, 103, 107, 108, 109, 110, 111, 112, 113, 114, 115, 116, 117, 118, 128, 133, 134, 138, 140, 141, 144, 145
classification PLA, 138
composite carriers, 2, 17

D

DNA-hybrid materials, 40
drug release system, 95, 100, 101, 108, 109

E

electrospinning cellulose acetate (CA), 12, 27, 35, 47
enzyme, 7, 8, 9, 10, 11, 12, 13, 14, 15, 16, 17, 18, 25, 26, 27, 28, 29, 47, 159

F

food packaging, 6, 76, 77, 78, 86, 120

G

gelatin, 10, 11, 24, 28, 53, 54, 55, 56, 57, 58, 59, 60, 61, 62, 63, 64, 65, 66, 67, 68, 69, 70, 71, 72, 73, 133, 143, 144

I

immobilisation methods, 2

L

lignin, viii, ix, 46, 147, 148, 149, 150, 151, 152, 153, 154, 155, 156, 157, 158, 159,
160, 161, 162, 163, 164, 165, 166, 167, 168, 169

M

modification of polymers, 2, 23
Molybdenum disulfide (MoS_2)/polyvinyl alcohol (PVA), viii, 119, 120, 121, 122, 123, 124, 125, 126, 127, 128, 129, 130, 131, 132, 134

N

nanocomposites, 20, 31, 32, 33, 34, 35, 36, 37, 38, 39, 40, 41, 42, 43, 44, 45, 46, 47, 48, 49, 50, 51, 66, 75, 76, 77, 78, 79, 80, 82, 84, 85, 86, 87, 88, 89, 90, 91, 92, 93, 94, 95, 103, 104, 106, 110, 112, 116, 118, 119, 120, 121, 122, 123, 124, 125, 126, 127, 128, 129, 130, 131, 132, 133, 134, 135, 136
nanomaterial, 43, 95
non-toxic and biocompatible, 128

O

osteoconductive scaffolds, 127

P

Pectin, 6, 140
pharmaceutical, 6, 32, 40, 41, 44, 53, 55, 100, 105
polylactide (PLA), 5, 20, 21, 22, 57, 75, 76, 77, 78, 79, 80, 81, 82, 83, 84, 85, 86, 87, 89, 90, 91, 92, 94, 138, 139
polymer, 2, 4, 6, 8, 9, 10, 11, 13, 14, 15, 19, 21, 23, 25, 26, 27, 32, 33, 35, 36, 37, 38, 39, 43, 50, 55, 56, 58, 60, 76, 77, 78, 80, 84, 87, 91, 96, 101, 102, 103, 104, 115,

116, 119, 120, 121, 122, 129, 138, 140, 147, 148, 150, 152, 158, 162, 166, 167
polysaccharides, 2, 5, 6, 35, 95, 96, 97, 98, 99, 100, 105, 106, 138, 140, 163
polyvinyl alcohol (PVA), 103, 119, 120, 121, 122, 123, 124, 125, 126, 127, 128, 129, 130, 131, 132, 134
properties, 2, 3, 6, 10, 13, 14, 15, 16, 17, 19, 20, 22, 27, 28, 32, 33, 34, 38, 39, 42, 43, 44, 45, 46, 47, 50, 52, 53, 56, 57, 58, 61, 62, 63, 67, 71, 76, 77, 78, 79, 80, 84, 86, 87, 90, 92, 93, 96, 97, 101, 103, 104, 107, 109, 110, 113, 120, 123, 125, 126, 127, 129, 131, 132, 133, 135, 136, 137, 138, 139, 141, 143, 144, 145, 147, 152, 153, 163, 164, 166

PVA/MMT nanocomposites, 121, 125

T

tissue engineering, x, 3, 6, 8, 24, 41, 53, 54, 55, 57, 59, 62, 64, 65, 66, 68, 69, 71, 72, 77, 84, 86, 102, 120, 126, 127, 130, 138, 141

tissue scaffolding, 42, 127

W

water-soluble polymer, 129
wound healing, ix, 8, 61, 64, 69, 130, 138, 142

Related Nova Publications

THE CRISPR/CAS9 SYSTEM: APPLICATIONS AND TECHNOLOGY

EDITOR: Alfred A. Bertelsen

SERIES: Biochemistry and Molecular Biology in the Post Genomic Era

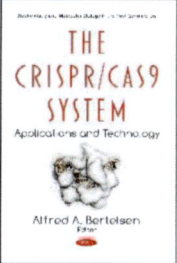

BOOK DESCRIPTION: This compilation focuses on the CRISPR/Cas9 system, a genome editing tool that has been hailed as the most profound molecular biology discovery in the past decade.

SOFTCOVER ISBN: 978-1-53616-426-8
RETAIL PRICE: $95

TREHALOSE: SOURCES, CHEMISTRY AND APPLICATIONS

EDITORS: Elżbieta Łopieńska-Biernat and Robert Stryiński

SERIES: Biochemistry and Molecular Biology in the Post Genomic Era

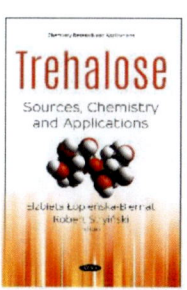

BOOK DESCRIPTION: Considering both the advantages and disadvantages of this sugar for humans, *Trehalose: Sources, Chemistry and Applications* emphasizes the importance of trehalose in both basic and applied research and presents an overview of its biological significance.

SOFTCOVER ISBN: 978-1-53614-944-9
RETAIL PRICE: $95

To see a complete list of Nova publications, please visit our website at www.novapublishers.com